The Race
Set Before Us

The Race
Set Before Us

Ken Radke

Thomas Nelson Publishers
Nashville

Published in Nashville, Tennessee, by Thomas Nelson, Inc. and distributed in Canada by Lawson Falle, Ltd., Cambridge, Ontario.

Printed in the United States of America

Unless otherwise indicated, Scripture quotations are from the *New American Standard Bible*, © The Lockman Foundation 1960, 1962, 1963, 1968, 1971, 1972, 1973, 1975 and are used by permission.

Scripture quotations marked NIV are taken from the Holy Bible: New International Version. Copyright © 1978 by the New York International Bible Society. Used by permission of Zondervan Bible Publishers.

The Scripture quotations marked PHILLIPS are taken from J. B. Phillips: THE NEW TESTAMENT IN MODERN ENGLISH, Revised Edition. © J. B. Phillips 1958, 1960, 1972. Used by permission of Macmillan Publishing Co., Inc.

The Scripture quotation marked RSV is from the Revised Standard Version of the Bible, copyrighted 1946, 1952, © 1971, 1973.

The Scripture quotation marked NKJB is from the New King James Bible— New Testament. Copyright © 1979, Thomas Nelson, Inc.

Photographs in this book are by David L. Kyle and Ron Anderson and are used by permission.

To my father, Henry Radke,
who at seventy-three years of age
still runs five miles a day
and sets a good example
for his sons.

Introduction

There is a race that is set before every person. This race involves living a life that is both pleasing to God and useful to people. The course has already been marked out for us. There are definite rules to be kept. There are specific obstacles to be avoided. There are training patterns to be practiced. There are successful runners to serve as models, and defeated runners to serve as warnings.

All this coaching is found in God's word—the Bible. In it we are instructed to "run with endurance the race that is set before us, fixing our eyes on Jesus, the author and perfecter of faith. . ." (Heb. 12:1,2). Some are just getting started in their run of faith. Many have already completed the course successfully and won the prize.

Jesus Christ invites every person to participate. As the God-man, He is no armchair spectator. He has lived where we live; He has been tempted as we are tempted. Yet He lived a sinless life and, having died for the sins of the world, cried out, "It is finished." By His resurrection He was the first to cross the finish line. He offers new life and strength to everyone who will follow Him.

This book is written for those with a love for running. It is *not* an encouragement to greater physical fitness. Rather, it shows how the passages in the Bible that deal with running and fitness relate to developing a strong spiritual life. The Bible doesn't push running and fitness. Rather, it assumes that people exercise, run, and compete, and it draws from these practices to exhort us to greater godliness.

We live in an age when all the major issues of life are reversed. The order of priorities for modern man is body, soul, then spirit (a distant third). God reverses the order.

"May your spirit and soul and body be preserved complete, without blame at the coming of our Lord Jesus Christ" (1 Thess. 5:23). These pages are devoted to helping us establish those priorities.

The book is set up as a devotional guide with questions at the end of each reading. A time of daily Bible study and prayer is recommended. This guide has fifty-two readings, so one reading could be used at the beginning of each week. The reader may want to read, meditate on, and then pray over each devotional. This could be done in as little as ten to fifteen minutes. To get the most benefit from each reading, time should be spent praying about applying the principles to your life.

Just as unused muscles seem to resent our first efforts at exercise, so our spirits will sometimes resist changes in character. But as we trust in Christ, He will give us the motivation and power to change. New acts of obedience may be difficult at first, but as spiritual muscles are used they become strong.

It is my prayer that each person who uses this book will be strengthened in his faith in Jesus Christ and be better equipped to run the race that is set before him.

I would like to thank my wife, Sue, for her invaluable help in expressing ideas intelligently; my friend, Bill Long, for examples from the running world; and a great mother-in-law, Meta Young, for her help in typing.

The Race
Set Before Us

1. Keeping Perspective

Train yourself in godliness; for while bodily training is of some value, godliness is of value in every way, as it holds promise for the present life and also for the life to come (1 Tim. 4:7,8 RSV).

A well-known running authority has said, "To run is life itself!" Many dedicated runners have been concerned by such statements and by the religious fervor that some attach to running and physical fitness. For many, running has become their religion, their God. But the Christian knows that only Jesus Christ is worthy of first place in his life. Paul wrote, "For to me, to live is Christ" (Phil. 1:21).

Believers realize that their bodies are temples of the Holy Spirit, and that they should take good care of them. But they also realize that their spirits are of far greater value, because their spirits live forever. Therefore, physical training is valuable, but training in godliness is even better. Godliness, or God-likeness, is the goal of the Christian life. Paul said, "I run in such a way, as not without aim. . . . I press on toward the goal . . ." (1 Cor. 9:26; Phil. 3:14). For Paul, becoming Christlike in his character was a goal worthy of striving toward.

Dr. Kenneth Cooper, an advocate of preventive medicine, has said that the fit person is the person with the best heart. Studies have proved the clear relationship between physical fitness and a strong cardiovascular system.

Solomon said, "Watch over your heart with all diligence, for from it flow the springs of life" (Prov. 4:23). All the issues of life are determined in one's heart. Therefore, spiritual training should be aimed at producing Christlike heart attitudes such as purity, honesty, humility, gratefulness, and love.

Physical training may result in a longer life, but spiritual training in godliness will produce a life pleasing to God.

Do you have a program for training in godliness?

How can you get started?

2. Living Within Boundaries

If anyone competes as an athlete, he does not win the prize unless he competes according to the rules (2 Tim. 2:5).

Our high school had an underground track in the basement, carved out among pillars that held up the building. There were eleven laps to a mile. Among the distance runners were Rich and Bob, identical twins who were quite good. Once, Rich was participating in a mile race. After about a half mile, Rich looked very tired and fell back from first place to last. But soon he came back to first place, looking as fresh as if he had just started.

Of course, it wasn't Rich at all. Bob had hidden behind a pillar and exchanged places with him after half a mile. They won, but they did not receive the "victor's crown" after their caper was discovered.

A man must compete according to rules in the spiritual realm as well. God has given us commands that are to be obeyed. Those who follow these commands will receive a spiritual crown at the end of their days. In an age when people are seeking to bend the rules, we need to develop the attitude of David, the great king of Israel, who said, "I shall run the way of Thy commandments" (Ps. 119:32). We must run the race of our daily lives within confines of the moral standards God has set for us in the Bible, that we may be rewarded at the end of the race.

Are you committed to living within the boundaries God has set for your life through His commands?

3. The Impossible Dream

. . . Christ in you, the hope of glory (Col. 1:27).

Suppose you were a runner of average ability who longed to be a world-class runner. But even with the most positive attitude and the best training program, your fastest time only put you near the middle of the pack. Then one night you dreamed that all of the ability, mental outlook, speed, endurance, and training of Bill Rodgers, the world-famous marathoner, came into you. In your dream you retained your own mind, will, personality, physical appearance, and even weaknesses, but within you were all of Bill Rodgers's strengths. Now, in your dream, you began to win races in world-record times. Everyone crowded around you, asking for your secret.

This impossible dream comes true in the spiritual life of every child of God. But instead of gaining the strengths of a famous runner, the Christian receives the strengths of Jesus Christ Himself! When Christ comes into a person's heart, He doesn't bypass his personality or cause his weaknesses to disappear. Christ doesn't overpower a person's will or give him unlimited success in every venture. Rather, He makes all the divine resources of God available to that person.

The apostle Paul put it this way: "In Him all the fulness of Deity dwells in bodily form, and in Him you have been made complete" (Col. 2:9,10). This means that God's wisdom, power, and love are available to a person through Christ. "God willed to make known what is the riches of the glory of this mystery among the Gentiles, which is Christ in you, the hope of glory" (Col. 1:27). A Christian is someone in whom Christ lives.

This mystery, or secret, is the impossible dream come true. It means that someone much greater than ourselves has come to live inside us. Christ desires to live His life through us, using us as His body to accomplish God's purposes on earth. We are living by the strength of another, One whose strength far transcends our own (2 Cor. 4:7).

To experience Christ's life in us, we must first know the reality of death to self. Paul wrote, "I have been crucified with Christ; and it is no longer I who live, but Christ lives in me" (Gal. 2:20). Whenever Paul felt the surge of his old ways taking over, he "died" to those urges. In the same way we can say, "Lord, in myself I will be irritable in this situation (or angry, depressed, etc.). But to the best of my ability I'm putting that to death right now. Cause Your patience to flow through me." Then we simply trust Him in confidence to do it.

Everything we lack and everything we need can be found in Christ. He lives through Joni Eareckson in a wheelchair. He lived through Corrie ten Boom in a Nazi prison camp. He lived through Elisabeth Elliott as she ministered to the Indians in Equador who had killed her husband. He lived through Hudson Taylor as he pioneered missionary work in inland China.

Our situation may not be as difficult as any of those. Yet we often find ourselves falling so far short in our ability to cope with our responsibilities that we cry out with Paul, "Who is adequate for these things?" (2 Cor. 2:16). The answer is that we have an all-sufficient Savior who is able to make us sufficient (see 2 Cor. 3:5,6). He is able to meet every one of our needs with His unlimited resources. In Christ are hidden all the treasures of wisdom (see Col. 2:3). He has been given all power and authority in both heaven and earth. (see Matt. 28:18). He is the one who loved us to the point of dying for us (see Eph. 5:2).

Leave your life of poverty and let Christ make you rich with His character. His way is not a life of passivity or ease but one of active trust in Him. It ends any boasting in our own puny efforts and begins a life of praise for His mighty works in and through us (1 Cor. 1:30,31).

What self-centered reactions need to die in order for you to experience more of Christ?

Reflect on the thought, "I live by faith in the Son of God" (Gal. 2:20). Is this true of you?

4. Renewed Strength

He gives strength to the weary, and to him who lacks might He increases power. Though youths grow weary and tired, and vigorous young men stumble badly, yet those who wait for the LORD will gain new strength; they will mount up with wings like eagles, they will run and not get tired, they will walk and not become weary (Is. 40:29–31).

Rudy Chapel, a high school runner with exceptional ability, was seeking to qualify for the 1976 Olympic tryouts. It seemed that if ever there were a high school student who could qualify for the 10,000-meters, Rudy was the one. He was running a good race until he was overcome by exhaustion. He slowed to such a snail's pace that his final quarter mile was almost a walk.

Rudy's run is a picture of what many are experiencing today in the race of life. They are overcome by demanding jobs, stress-filled homes, and the pressures of daily life. They fall victim to weariness. Many, even strong young men, stumble and fall. Like Rudy Chapel, they have slowed to a snail's pace and are at the point of sheer exhaustion.

It is to this type of person that Isaiah addresses his encouragement. Only the weak and weary qualify, because they are the ones who recognize their need for God's strength and power. Jim Ryun, a one-time world-record holder in the half mile and 1500 meters, used to train himself to sprint when he was exhausted. This training method carried him to three Olympic Games. So too, a Christian can train himself to meet emotional and spiritual weariness by depending on God's strength in the hour of testing.

Isaiah says, "They will run and not get tired." The key to

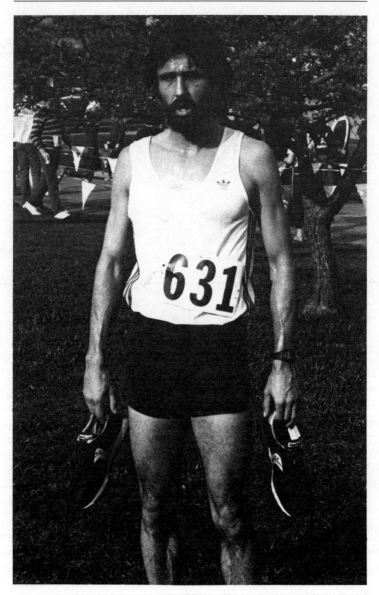

living without weariness is to hope in, or wait upon, the Lord. By turning to Him at each point of weakness and laying the situation before Him, we have access to His inexhaustible supply of power and strength. "Lord, I can't handle this. My strength is gone. But Your power is unlimited and You can handle it. Thank You." Only the person who lives by God's strength will be able to "run and not get tired."

Paul said, "When I am weak, then I am strong" (2 Cor. 12:10). It is at our point of weakness that we are motivated to call out for the strength of another. And His strength is freely available to all who "wait for the Lord."

What factors are producing weariness in your life?

How can you renew your strength?

5. The Narrow Road

I shall run the way of Thy commandments (Ps. 119:32).

King David excelled as a poet, a musician, a preacher, a military strategist, and a moral and political leader of his nation. The secret behind his greatness was not his gifts, but his character. He was an extremely obedient man. When he chose to disobey God by committing adultery with Bathsheba, his leadership began to slip. Yet through God's forgiveness and mercy he remained the greatest king in Israel's history. David was a great runner who followed the path of God's commands.

There are two factors in David's obedience. The first is that he ran to perform God's commands. Many obey God, but only after much delay and procrastination. Delayed obedience is actually disobedience. God is looking for people who, as soon as they know what God wants of them, run quickly to do it. Obedience has been defined as "doing what God says to do, right away, with the right heart attitude." David ran quickly to obey God.

The second factor in David's obedience is that he pursued God's path. The Bible speaks of two roads: the broad, easy way and the narrow, difficult way. God's way is often the difficult road.

When I was in high school trying to make the two-mile relay team, I hurt my ankle running the turns on the small banked track. The doctor said I could continue running straightaways, but no turns for a month. So I ran alone in a nearby park, battling cold weather and hills. This "narrow, difficult road" proved better for developing my speed than the warm indoor track. When I returned after a month, I easily made the team.

Jesus said, "The way is broad that leads to destruction, and many are those who enter by it. . . . The way is narrow that leads to life, and few are those who find it" (Matt. 7:13,14). The majority of people are not running on the narrow road, but if you choose it you'll be in good company.

To stay on the "narrow road" is to live inside the boundary lines God has established for your life. Often this involves living by a higher standard than those around us. One man's motto is, "Others may, but I may not." It may mean not dating a non-Christian, refusing to go to certain types of entertainment, or limiting your freedom in other ways, so that you are sure to stay inside God's boundary lines. To others, this may appear narrow-minded, old-fashioned, or negative. But to the Spirit-led Christian it is a way of joy, because it is God's way and He is the Source of all true joy.

"The lines have fallen to me in pleasant places; Indeed, my heritage is beautiful to me. . . . Thou wilt make known to me the path of life; In Thy presence is fulness of joy; In Thy right hand there are pleasures forever (Ps. 16:6,11).

What boundary lines has God set for you?

Are you joyfully running on that narrow road?

6. Personalized Fitness

When they measure themselves by themselves, and compare themselves with themselves, they are without understanding (2 Cor. 10:12).

Many young people pattern themselves after famous athletes, trying to copy their styles, diets, attitudes, and training programs. To a certain extent this is good as it provides the youngsters with successful models and a certain amount of motivation. But it can also be very dangerous and limiting.

Each of us has been given unique gifts and abilities. We cannot live up to someone else's abilities but only to our own. A particular training program may have taken Frank Shorter to the Olympics, but that same program could be totally wrong for someone else. Each person is different.

So it is in the spiritual life. A Christian can become discouraged when he sets his sights on becoming like some gifted person when he himself lacks those gifts. The opposite problem—self-satisfaction and pride—can arise when Christians compare themselves to others who are like them, as the Corinthians did. Using themselves as the standard of comparison, the Corinthians all came out smelling like roses! But Paul had to remind them that their whole church at Corinth was substandard. He had to rebuke them, saying, "I, brethren, could not speak to you as to spiritual men, but as to men of the flesh, as to babes in Christ" (1 Cor. 3:1). So we see that comparing can lead to discouragement or to arrogance.

The particular spiritual training program one Christian follows may not be right for another. Martin Luther arose each day at four in the morning to pray, but that does not mean all Christians should do the same. A respected spiritual leader may exercise the freedom to follow a particular lifestyle, but that lifestyle may not be right for every Christian. God has a particular training program for each person.

I once heard a man give a message on the importance of having devotions as soon as one gets out of bed each morning. God led him to make the vow, "No Bible, no breakfast!" He tried to get his audience to make that same vow. I did not. Although I have my devotions before breakfast 95 percent of the time, I want to follow my own convictions, not another man's.

If you are a teachable disciple, you will study the lives of great Christians and observe carefully the example of godly believers around you. You will allow yourself to be challenged and motivated by others. Yet you will avoid both discouragement and arrogance, because other people are not your ultimate model. God is the only model wholly worth imitating. Rather than looking to people, you will look to Christ. Then you can say, with Paul, "We all, . . . beholding as in a mirror the glory of the Lord, are being transformed into the same image from glory to glory" (2 Cor. 3:18). As you look to Christ, you become like Him.

Sometimes we are tempted to look at others and say, "But Lord, you seem to be so lenient on them and so hard on me!" Peter had this same problem when he asked, "Lord, what about him?" (referring to John).

Jesus answered him, "What is that to you? You follow Me!" (John 21:21,22).

As a Christian, I have one Lord in my life—Jesus Christ. My only job is to look to Him in faith and follow His personalized instructions for me.

In what areas do you compare yourself with others spiritually?

What personal convictions have you developed directly from God's Word?

7. Stay on the Right Course

It was because of a revelation that I went up; and I submitted to them the gospel which I preach . . . for fear that I might be running, or had run, in vain (Gal. 2:2).

I once observed a local six-mile race where the course was not marked very clearly. In the last half mile, the two leading runners each took a different route to the finish line. One of them made a wrong turn, and his whole race was run in vain.

Paul was concerned that the Galatians were doing that same thing. He first showed them that he had checked out the gospel of salvation by faith alone with the Jerusalem church leaders (see Gal. 2:2). Then he showed the Galatians that they had abandoned this gospel of faith in Christ by requiring certain works. He bluntly questioned them: "You were running well; who hindered you from obeying the truth?" (Gal. 5:7).

We begin the Christian life by putting our faith in Christ and receiving Him into our hearts. The Galatians had done this. We continue living the Christian life by faith. This is where the Galatians erred. They began to put their trust in religious works, such as circumcision. We cannot earn our way to heaven. Only Jesus can take us there.

Like the six-mile runner, many people today have begun their Christian life the right way but are living it the wrong way. They must answer the question Paul asked the Galatians, "Are you so foolish? Having begun by the Spirit, are you now being perfected by the flesh?" (Gal. 3:3). The Christian life is not only difficult; it is humanly impossible. It can only be lived by faith in what Christ has done for us and is doing in us.

Have you been routed off the faith course onto the human effort course?

How can you tell whether you are living by faith or by human effort and self-trust?

24

8. Rest and Work

There remains therefore a Sabbath rest for the people of God. For the one who has entered His rest has himself also rested from his works, as God did from His (Heb. 4:9,10).

Derek Clayton, a former world-record holder in the marathon, has said that to be relaxed is the most important aspect of running a good time in a race. In training patterns, many runners practice a hard—easy cycle: one day for long, hard mileage with speed followed by a day of easy, light mileage. It is during the "resting" times that the muscle tissue rebuilds itself and becomes stronger. In the spiritual life there are two rests to be entered.

The first is the rest of salvation, when we stop trusting in our own work to get us to heaven. Christ's death on the cross secures heaven for us, and we can rest in that finished work. This rest begins the moment we place our faith in Christ.

The second rest is to be lived out moment by moment in our daily lives. It is the rest of faith, trusting God to work in us and through us. Only through this rest can we avoid the exhaustion and weariness that plagues so many of us in this fast-paced society. Only by resting in Christ can we live our lives in a relaxed way, free of exhaustion.

Jesus Christ promised us this rest, when He said, "Come to Me, all who are weary and heavy-laden, and I will give you rest. Take My yoke upon you, and learn from Me, for I am gentle and humble in heart; and you shall find rest for your souls" (Matt. 11:28,29). This promise of rest has only two conditions. First, we must come to Jesus when we feel exhausted. Second, we must take His yoke upon us, making Him our Lord and Teacher and letting Him decide what we should or should not do.

Our burdens are often heavy and unbearable. We see an

exhausted businessman bringing home a pile of work, a weary mother trudging through the grocery store with a child hanging on each of her legs. Jesus Christ promised that His yoke is easy and His burden light (see Matt. 11:30). But where is the rest for these overworked and exhausted people?

The key is to allow Jesus Christ to be Lord. This means letting Him set up our schedule and tell us what to do *and what not to do*. There will always be time and energy to do His will. It is when we try to live up to other's expectations, or our own unrealistic standards, that we get into trouble. Our burden is heavy. His burden is light.

At the end of Christ's three-year ministry He said to God the Father, "I glorified Thee on the earth, having accomplished the work which Thou hast given Me to do" (John 17:4). Jesus didn't accomplish all the work there was in the world, but He did finish everything His Father assigned to Him. Christ was submitted fully to the lordship of the Father, just as we are to be to the lordship of the Son.

Oswald Chambers has said of God's will, "His calling is His enablement." If you have two very dependent toddlers, then He will give you the strength to cope. If He has called you to a high-pressure job, to teach a Sunday school class, and to serve on two committees, then He will strengthen you to do each one well.

The apostle Paul knew the secret of strenuous hard work carried out with a peaceful attitude of rest. He wrote, "Work out your salvation with fear and trembling, for it is God who is at work in you" (Phil. 2:12,13). When Jesus Christ is Lord and Master, we will know the secret of letting Him direct our activities and energize us to accomplish them. Then we will be able to work to our fullest capacity, while at the same time relaxing in His adequacy.

Can you say with confidence that Christ is the Lord of your life and that He is the one who orders your schedule?

Are you overcommitted or just under-empowered?

9. Heavenly Grandstands

Therefore, since we have so great a cloud of witnesses surrounding us, let us . . . run with endurance the race that is set before us (Heb. 12:1).

In high school, as a member of our four-mile relay team, I participated in one of the biggest relays in the state. The stands were filled. On the last lap of my mile run, I passed the lead runner and handed the baton to my teammate. Our team won the race and set a new school record. But that honor meant little compared to what happened just after I finished my part of the relay. As I was walking, exhausted, next to the crowded stands, a hand reached out to me. I looked up and saw the smiling, proud face of my dad. I'll never forget the joy of that moment.

The Book of Hebrews tells us that we are running our race of faith before a heavenly grandstand. All the believers who have lived and died make up the "great cloud of witnesses." Not only are they cheering for us, but their lives are models for us to follow. Knowing of their successes can spur us on to greater victories. Hebrews 11 lists "faith's hall of fame"—people who were commended for their faith. Then in Hebrews 12 the writer says we are surrounded by these witnesses, people who put their trust in a trustworthy God. Abel ran the race; Enoch ran the race; Noah ran the race; Abraham ran the race—and they all finished successfully by trusting in God.

You, too, can finish the race by trusting in that same God. Don't give up! Remember the witnesses sitting in the grandstands. Many of them were ordinary people just like you. They trusted in God, and He helped them to finish the race.

Someday each of us who has lived faithfully will meet

those in the grandstand and share with them the joy of having completed the race successfully.

Do you live your life with an awareness that all of heaven observes your actions?

In what issues of your life have you proved, along with Noah, Abraham, and others, that God is trustworthy?

10. Avoiding the Rocks

*Keep faith and a good conscience, which some have re-
jected and suffered shipwreck in regard to their faith
(1 Tim. 1:19).*

Every athlete must avoid some pitfalls. It may be arguing
with an official, losing one's temper, losing one's concentra-
tion, or perhaps overtraining. But for a sailor, the greatest
danger is the rocks. Many a ship has strayed from the center
of the channel or gone too close to the shore and suffered
destruction on jagged rocks.

A Christian can also become shipwrecked. The spiritual life
is not always smooth sailing, and there are dangers to be
avoided. Foolhardy sailors will see how close they can get to
the danger without crashing. The *Titanic* sailed through a
dangerous area at fast speeds. Many Christians have taken a
similar course, with tragic results. Paul described some people in New Testament times who rejected "good conscience."
In ignoring that inner voice, they veered toward the rocks.
They continued to practice things they knew were wrong and
turned a deaf ear to the voice of conscience. Before long they
hit the rocks, shattering their faith in God and ruining their
spiritual lives. Those who ignore warnings always pay the
price.

Just as a wise sailor will steer well clear of the rocks, so a
wise Christian will seek to stay far away from sin and make no
compromises with his conscience. Conscience is not the abso-
lute guide for right and wrong, but we are never free to
ignore or reject it.

A diligent sailor works hard at keeping his ship on course.
To do so requires strength, endurance, alertness, and skill.
His eyes constantly watch the water, and he is fully aware of

his charts. In like manner, the diligent Christian navigates carefully around obstacles, keeping a sharp eye on the path he is pursuing. When his conscience rebukes him, he immediately stops the activity he is pursuing and follows a different course.

The Ten Commandments speak to black-and-white issues, but the conscience speaks to issues in the gray area. Whoever wants to avoid spiritual shipwreck remembers that "All things are lawful for me, but not all things are profitable" (1 Cor. 6:12).

Do you know any people who have made a shipwreck of their spiritual lives?

Pray that God would give you a greater alertness to the dangers near you.

11. Stumbling

When you walk, your steps will not be impeded; and if you run, you will not stumble (Prov. 4:12).

To run without stumbling is the desire of every runner. This verse from the Book of Proverbs tells us this is possible if we listen carefully to God's words and follow His instructions. But none of us does that perfectly. Everyone stumbles and falls, but some never get up again. Stumbling is not the problem. Failure to get up is the problem.

Jim Ryun, a great distance runner, had difficulty with stumbling. Because of an inner ear problem, he sometimes lost his balance and fell down. Jim could have been destroyed by this problem, but he won races in spite of it.

Lasse Viren, from Finland, was competing in the finals of the 10,000 meters at the 1972 Olympic Games. Seconds after the gun sounded to start the race, Lasse fell! It was like a nightmare. A man who had hoped to win the race was on the ground! He sat there for a moment and then bounced up. By this time the best runners had opened up a large lead, but Lasse was determined not to give up. He caught up with the leaders, passed them, and won the gold medal.

The Scriptures show the same pattern of perseverance. Solomon said, "A righteous man falls seven times, and rises again" (Prov. 24:16). Micah said, "Though I fall I will rise" (Mic. 7:8). Paul said, "We may be knocked down but we are never knocked out!" (2 Cor. 4:9 PHILLIPS). All these passages picture a runner who falls, even as many as seven times, but who always picks himself up to get back in the race.

Perhaps a person fails in business, in family leadership, or in personal morality. Each time there is a failure, a person must decide: will I give up or will I get up? Someone has said,

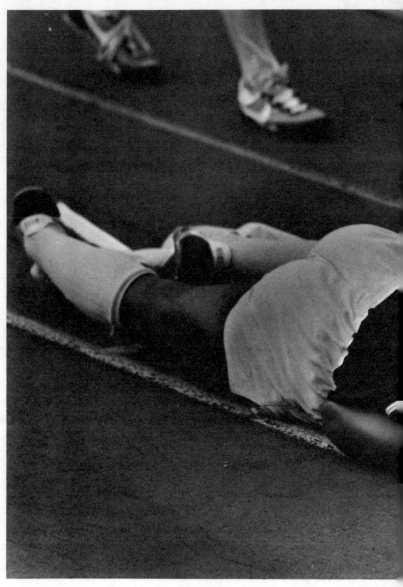

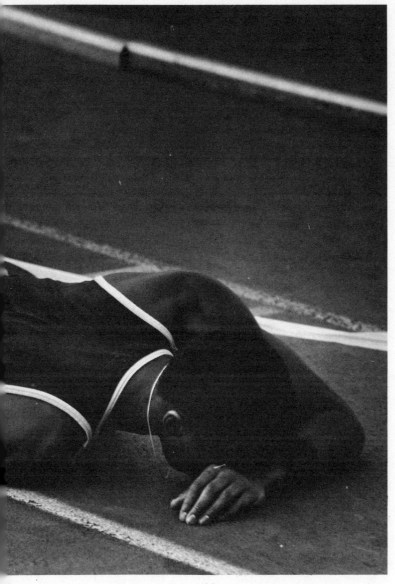

"A failure is not someone who fails. A failure is someone who fails and gives up." There is a difference between experiencing some failings and becoming a failure.

Once a person has learned that he must get up after he falls, then he is ready to learn the second great lesson. "[He] is able to keep you from stumbling . . ." (Jude 24). This is the foundational truth supporting the statement that "when you run, you will not stumble."

Jesus Christ ran the race before me and never fell once, and He is able to keep me from falling. He will protect me by two things. First, I am protected by His powerful Word. As I listen to it, quote it, and obey it, I will be kept from falling. Second, I am protected by the humility He produces in me. It has been said, "He who will not be humble will stumble." Humility enables me to remember the times I've fallen in the past, thereby keeping me alert for any potential stumblings. Scripture says, "Pride goes before destruction, and a haughty spirit before stumbling" (Prov. 16:18).

The apostle Paul was a man who remembered his past failures, and doing so kept him humble and upright to run the race set before him. ". . . even though I was formerly a blasphemer and a persecutor and a violent aggressor. And yet I was shown mercy, because I acted ignorantly and in unbelief; and the grace of our Lord was more than abundant, with the faith and love which are found in Christ Jesus" (1 Tim. 1:13,14).

How do you react when you fail?

What attitude should you take when you fail?

12. Heat

When I kept silent about my sin, my body wasted away through my groaning all day long. For day and night Thy hand was heavy upon me; my vitality was drained away as with the fever-heat of summer. I acknowledged my sin to Thee, and my iniquity I did not hide; I said, "I will confess my transgressions to the Lord"; and Thou didst forgive the guilt of my sin (Ps. 32:3–5).

It was a hot, humid day in August of 1978 for the running of the Falmouth Road race. Alberto Salazar, a world-class distance runner, crossed the finish line in tenth place and then passed out. He was immediately taken to the hospital and packed in ice as his blood pressure dropped, his temperature climbed, and he went into convulsions. He was a victim of heatstroke. Runners are able to endure cold and snow, rain and hail, but heat is the most serious threat to their health and life. Alberto recovered, but without quick medical attention the story might have ended differently.

Because of sin, the world has become a hot, dry place to live. David prayed, "My soul thirsts for Thee, my flesh yearns for Thee, in a dry and weary land where there is no water" (Ps. 63:1). But our surroundings are not all that is hot and dry. Sometimes we are, too. David spoke of his own strength being drained, as on a sweltering summer day. This was caused by a failure to confess his sins to God.

All people sin (see Rom. 3:23). Confession is to the spirit what sweating is to the body. When our bodies overheat, we sweat. The body's heat is carried to the skin through the blood. There the sweat evaporates, cooling the blood. A person who doesn't sweat adequately will overheat. In the same way, our spirits will overheat unless our sin is brought to the

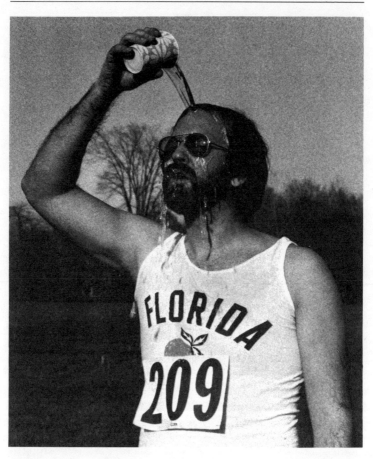

surface and released by admitting to God that we are guilty
and asking for forgiveness. As we practice this regularly, we
will be cleansed and freed from guilt.

Jesus Christ took the penalty of our sin and provided forgiveness for us when He died on the cross (see Is. 53:4–6). But
if we don't admit that we've sinned, then our sins will produce bitterness and guilt in our lives, and our spiritual
strength will be drained. But if we confess our sins quickly

and specifically to God, we will know and experience His wonderful forgiveness (see 1 John 1:9).

This is the promise of God to the humble, repentant person: "Though your sins are as scarlet, they will be as white as snow" (Is. 1:18). When David confessed his adultery, he took the promise one step further: "Purify me with hyssop, and I shall be clean; wash me, and I shall be whiter than snow" (Ps. 51:7). No sin is too great that it cannot be forgiven and cleansed by the blood of Christ (see 1 John 1:7). In God's sight, the dark stains of our sin are cleansed and we shine like the brightness of new-fallen snow on a sunny day.

Just as heat is the most serious threat to a runner's physical health, so sin is the most serious threat to a Christian's spiritual health. But through the conviction of the Spirit, the confession of the believer, and the cleansing of the blood, there comes spiritual health and joy.

Make a list of any unconfessed sins and ask God's forgiveness now.

Believe that you are now whiter than snow in God's sight.

13. Injuries

Therefore, strengthen the hands that are weak and the knees that are feeble, and make straight paths for your feet, so that the limb which is lame may not be put out of joint, but rather be healed (Heb. 12:12,13).

Bill Rodgers had set an American record and was hoping to win a gold medal in the 1976 Olympics. But one month before the race, Bill hurt his foot and was not able to train properly. No one knew but his doctor. Although Bill was favored to win, he placed a disappointing twenty-fifth because of his injury. Every athlete hates injuries because they may ruin his career. Similarly, we dread "injuries" in the spiritual life. But sometimes it is God who sends the injury. The Bible calls this "discipline" or "chastisement." These are painful times, but in the long run they prove beneficial if we recognize that they come from God for our good. But only by responding properly to them will we actually reap the potential benefits. "All discipline for the moment seems not to be joyful, but sorrowful; yet to those who have been trained by it, afterwards it yields the peaceful fruit of righteousness" (Heb. 12:11).

The Greek word for "trained" gives us our English word "gymnasium." Many young people don't want to go to gym class. They don't want to change clothes, work, and sweat. In the spiritual realm, many don't want to submit to the spiritual gymnasium in order to be trained. They will learn from reading books or listening to sermons, but don't want to learn from the difficult experiences God sends their way. Yet God says, "Reproofs for discipline are the way of life" (Prov. 6:23).

The way to avoid future injuries is to strengthen yourself now. A person must humble himself first to recognize that God is disciplining him. He must take note of the specific area he has failed in and begin a program of strengthening himself in that area. If a runner has a weak knee, he must do exercises or receive therapy to build it up. If a Christian has a quick temper, or a critical spirit, or a selfish attitude, he must do spiritual exercises to build himself up in those areas.

The following three exercises, practiced frequently, are a wonderful way to build spiritual muscles. First, ask God each day to lead you in the opposite direction of temptation (see Matt. 6:13). Second, identify with Christ's death and resurrection by considering yourself dead to sin and alive to God. If your problem is a bad temper and God has been disciplining you for it, each time it wells up remind yourself that you are actually dead to that old way of living. Then consider yourself alive and responsive to God's new way of handling the problem through self-control. This is not mental gymnastics but living by spiritual realities (see Rom. 6:6,11). Third, praise God often that He is able to keep you from falling (see Jude 24).

These disciplines are the road to spiritual healing and health. Only those who practice them will avoid future injuries.

Are you aware of any discipline God is sending into your life to train you not to sin?

How can you benefit from this training?

14. The Masters

The glory of young men is their strength, and the honor of old men is their gray hair (Prov. 20:29).

So many older people are running today that race officials had to create a new category called the "masters" for competitors over forty. Not only have these runners reversed some of the deteriorating effects of aging and sedentary living, but many have shown surprising athletic ability. In 1975, Toronto hosted the first World Masters Track and Field Championship, where several hundred older people competed. Today, thousands are competing in races. In some major contests, more than half of the runners are over forty. My own father began running at sixty-five, and in the past ten years he has logged more than 3,900 miles.

Larry Lewis is remembered as one of the greatest older runners who ever performed. Beginning at age nine, he ran every day of his life until his death from cancer at age one hundred and six! His daily routine was to rise at four-thirty in the morning and run 6.7 miles. Then he would walk 5 miles to work, where he was a full-time waiter. Larry Lewis was one of the "masters."

This trend toward physical fitness among older people is commendable, and many more should be a part of it. Yet many older people are unable to be involved in such vigorous activity. Some are confined to wheelchairs, while others are hindered by arthritis or other physical problems.

Aging is feared by many people in our culture. Becoming older is difficult to accept when so much praise and worship is directed toward youthfulness. But God honors age and its accompanying wisdom. He declares gray hair to be the glory of an older person, not something to be hidden.

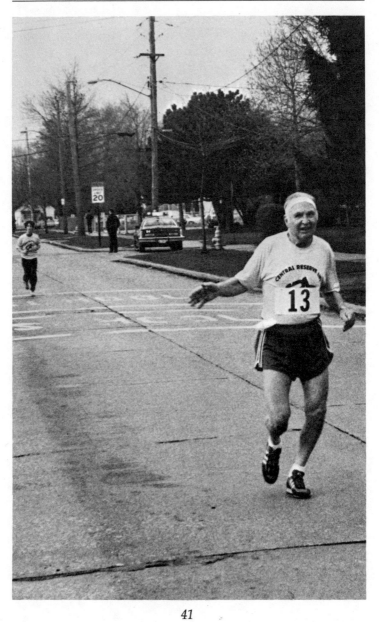

God's idea for perfection focuses not on the physical man, but on the hidden person of the heart. "Therefore we do not lose heart, but though our outer man is decaying, yet our inner man is being renewed day by day. . . . We look not at the things which are seen, but at the things which are not seen; For the things which are seen are temporal, but the things which are not seen are eternal" (2 Cor. 4:16,18).

The body will eventually die, but a man's spirit will live forever. When we experience that weakening process called aging, we need not become discouraged as long as we are growing spiritually. Every day our spirits can be renewed and become stronger and more beautiful. The growing Christian daily manifests more and more of God's strength and life.

Saints who have matured over the years become men and women of the Word of God. They become prayer warriors and accomplish great things for God through their faith. Even in old age they are still growing and bearing fruit (see Ps. 92:14). These people of God are examples to all who know them. They are God's "spiritual masters," and they realize that the best is yet to come.

Has aging brought any discouragement into your life?

How can this discouragement be counteracted?

15. Follow the Leader

Let us also lay aside every encumbrance, and the sin which so easily entangles us, and let us run with endurance the race that is set before us, fixing our eyes on Jesus, the author and perfecter of faith . . . (Heb. 12:1,2).

The Christian life is not a hundred-yard dash. It is far more like a distance run, full of hazards and requiring much endurance. In fact, the word "endure" is used four times in Hebrews 12. Endurance is the ability to withstand hardship or adversity over an extended period of time. That is far easier to do in the physical realm than it is in the spiritual realm. We often become weary and give up trying to live an effective Christian life.

The Christian needs the mindset of a distance runner who knows how to hold himself back at the beginning of the race and fight off weariness at the end. In the 1976 Olympics, a steeplechase runner was in second place coming into the final stretch. These contestants must jump over a series of barriers and a water hazard as they run the course. To a runner, it seems like the barriers get larger and larger as the race goes on. Out of sheer weariness, this second-place runner hit the last barrier, went down, and didn't even place in the race!

The author of this passage in Hebrews gives us two bits of spiritual counsel based on good running strategy. The first is to strip off every weight and sin—much as a runner would get rid of his sweat suit before the race or choose a light pair of shoes. Ridding our lives of sins and practices that are clearly wrong is obviously necessary. It's not easy, but it's essential. Persistent sin patterns will entangle our feet as surely as will a dog nipping at a jogger's heels. Once, two dogs came after me while I was out running. The owner of the dogs stood by

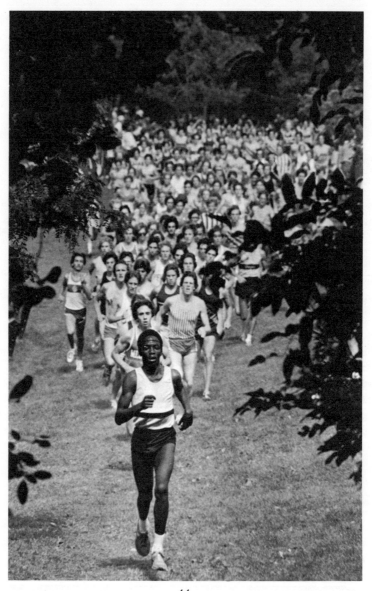

watching and said with a pleasant smile, "They like runners." It brought my run to a fast stop!

The writer of Hebrews also counsels us to rid ourselves of encumbrances or weights. "Weights" are practices that are not morally wrong, but that are slowing us down in the race. Once God impressed upon me that Monday Night Football was a weight in my life. It dominated my whole schedule and thought. Watching the game was a problem because my job required working evenings. I gave it up for a year and was happier because of doing so. Later, I was able to enjoy it without letting it dominate me.

The second word of counsel for running the Christian race is to "fix our eyes on Jesus." If a runner watches the ground it can have a hypnotic effect causing him to lose touch with the other runners. If he watches the spectators, he also will fall behind. The best strategy is to keep his eyes fixed on the leader of the race.

For us as Christians, Jesus is the leader who goes before us. He has already completed the course successfully, without sin. Yet He still leads the way for us. Our part is to follow closely, not running impatiently ahead nor falling far behind. If we look to the circumstances or to ourselves, we will surely be defeated. We must focus our faith and our mental attention on Him "who for the joy set before him endured the cross" (Heb. 12:2).

As we see Christ's perfect power, love, and wisdom, we will draw strength from Him, enabling us to run with endurance. The person who lives his life looking to Jesus trusts in the unlimited resources of our perfect Leader. As we find our own resources and strength failing, we turn our eyes from ourselves to Christ, gaining new strength to run the race.

What weights or sins in your life must be stripped off so that you can "run the race" unhindered?

How can you fix your eyes on Jesus?

16. "I'm Not Running on Sunday"

". . . Those who honor Me I will honor . . ." (1 Sam. 2:30).

Eric Liddell, the winner of a gold medal in the 1924 Paris Olympics, has come to the attention of many through the popular movie "Chariots of Fire." In his day he was the hero of all of Scotland, and his fame spread to many parts of the world. In a time when the Olympics were not as extravagant as they are today, what was it that elevated this man to such fame and popularity? Even after he left the sporting world to be a missionary in China, his popularity with the masses continued. How could someone living in far-off China continue to hold the respect of his countrymen? What is it that has drawn thousands in our own country to see a movie based on his life?

Eric Liddell had a conviction that it was wrong to engage in sports on Sunday. He lived by that conviction. A conviction is not just an opinion you hold intellectually but a principle you live by and are even willing to die for. When it was announced that the qualifying heats of the 100 meters were being held on a Sunday, Eric Liddell announced, "I am not running on a Sunday." He saw it as God's day, and nothing would change his mind. He wasn't belligerent or judgmental of others. He didn't make a big fuss over it. He just lived by his conviction. He was also willing to suffer for his principles. The press criticism and being called a traitor to his country hurt him deeply. Yet he knew that following his principles was more important. Having made his decision, he ran instead in the 400 meters, not his normal event, and crossed the finish line first with a new world-record time of 47.6.

Certainly Eric Liddell was a gifted athlete. Yet he was known to have a terrible style with his arms flinging wildly and his head looking up toward the sky as he ran. Just before he ran the 400 meters the British team's trainer slipped him a note with a quote from 1 Samuel 2:30 on it: "Those who honor me I will honor. . . ." God honored Eric for following his principles. Even though many people did not agree with or embrace Eric's principles, they respected him for living by them.

In Old Testament times, Daniel was a man of uncompromising conviction who knew how to stand alone for his principles. His normal practice was to pray three times a day. His enemies had a law passed that forbade anyone to pray to any other god except King Darius for thirty days. Daniel knew he must obey God rather than man and stuck by his normal practice of praying to the Lord three times a day. He paid the consequences and was thrown to the lions. But God honored Daniel and saved him.

Daniel was a man willing to live for his convictions and even to die for them. He knew how to stand alone against the social rejection of those who disliked his convictions. Jesus said, "Blessed are those who have been persecuted for the sake of righteousness, for theirs is the kingdom of heaven" (Matt. 5:10).

We need people today who are willing to live by their convictions. We need people who would rather lose their jobs or go to jail than to compromise their convictions.

You need to stick to your principles even when people ". . . say all kinds of evil against you falsely . . ." (Matt. 5:11). Like Eric Liddell, you must quietly and humbly do what you think is right.

What principles are you presently being tempted to compromise?

Are you convinced that God will honor you if you honor Him?

17. The Winning Attitude

But thanks be to God, who always leads us in His triumph in Christ (2 Cor. 2:14).

The runner who wins has learned the importance of a positive mental attitude. To succeed he must have confidence in himself and in his training program. Most importantly, he must expect to win.

Likewise, a successful and victorious Christian must have positive attitudes and thoughts. This is not the same as "the power of positive thinking," where a person repeats positive statements to himself and waits for a strange magic to overtake him and lead him to success. Rather, Christians are to be responsible toward God in their thoughts. Paul said, ". . . we are taking every thought captive to the obedience of Christ." (2 Cor. 10:5).

It has been said: "Sow a thought and reap an attitude; sow an attitude and reap a character; sow a character and reap a destiny." Everything, great or small, good or evil, begins with our thoughts. If we recognize that God wants to lead us to victory, this truth will affect our thought lives. Even defeats can be turned into victory if we learn from them.

Many runners—and Christians—despise the day of small things. A runner who never has won even a five-mile race dreams of winning the Boston Marathon. The Christian who reads the Bible once a week desires to impart deep spiritual insights to others. But it's the smaller battles that need to be won.

One of the "smaller battles" many Christians are engaged in today has to do with the place of television in their lives. Television has led the way in lowering moral standards in our society. We now allow images and language into our living rooms that would have shocked and disgusted us ten years ago. Yet, we are lured by the desire for "entertainment" and diversion, and we sit entranced by the images on the silver screen.

What we watch and how much we watch are constant concerns of serious Christians. If we lose this battle—which affects our attitudes and thought life in a subtle but dangerous way—we will lose bigger and more important battles outside our homes. If we already are controlled by television, we have lost the battle. David said, "I will walk within my house in the integrity of my heart. I will set no worthless thing before my eyes" (Ps. 101:2). Christians will win the battle with television if they make this same commitment.

There are many "small" battles that God wants us to win. The victorious Christian is one who progressively recognizes pockets of defeat in his life and then allows Christ to enable him to win a victory in that area. When we first acknowledge some besetting sin, we are tempted to say, "There is no hope." But if we really want to experience victory, then we can confidently claim the promise that ". . . the desire of the righteous will be granted" (Prov. 10:24). As we mentally take these steps of faith and commitment we will discover that God is leading us in the triumphal procession. We will have a winning attitude.

In what areas are you losing battles and experiencing defeat?

How can you become victorious?

18. A Good Injury

The sun rose upon him just as he crossed over Peniel, and he was limping on his thigh (Gen. 32:31).

Years ago a young boy suffered terrible burns from a kerosene fire in his one-room schoolhouse. The doctors felt that even if his legs could be saved, he would never walk again. His mother worked with him day after day, rubbing his legs with oil to help the scar tissue stay soft. Eventually he began to walk, and then even to run. One day, this same man set a world record of 4:07 for the mile and became one of the greatest milers of all time. Glenn Cunningham was his name. Clearly, it was the injury that stimulated his determination to overcome, which led to athletic success and greatness. In a sense, it was a good injury.

Hundreds of years ago, there lived a man whose whole character was built upon deceit. He cheated his own family and others, creating a growing number of enemies. One day God confronted this man in a wrestling match and asked him, "What is your name?" The man answered that his name was Jacob, which means "he deceives." For the first time, Jacob came to the end of himself and honestly admitted and confessed his sinful nature. It was at this time that God changed his name to Israel.

During the wrestling match, God touched Jacob's hip socket so that he limped. His hip was injured for life, but his spirit and character were transformed for eternity. The limp was a constant reminder to him that he must no longer trust in his own scheming but rely fully upon God. It would remind Israel that he was no longer Jacob. In a sense, it was a good injury.

A more up-to-date example is Joni Eareckson, who became

a quadriplegic through a swimming accident at age seventeen. Since Joni accepted her injury and yielded herself fully to God, she has grown in Christlike character in a way that she might never have if she had the use of all her limbs. God has used her injury not only to deepen her own character, but to prove to thousands that Jesus Christ can turn even the darkest sorrow into rejoicing. Her wheelchair has become a pulpit. Her many speaking opportunities and the movie about her life have brought many people to Christ. Joni is not able to run or swim or ride horseback. But she is able to grow in character and point others to Jesus Christ and His life-transforming power. In a sense, it was a good injury.

Can you see good developing from a physical injury or limitation you have?

Why is a person's spirit more important than the body?

19. Competition

And the rain descended, and the floods came, and the winds blew, and burst against that house; and yet it did not fall, for it had been founded upon the rock (Matt. 7:25).

People enter competitive races for many reasons, but the underlying motive is to see how good they really are. Workouts give some indication, but the race tells the story.

The ultimate test of fitness is the marathon—26 miles and 385 yards of grueling endurance. More than 50,000 men and women run in marathons each year. The most famous is the Boston marathon, which began in 1897 with 15 participants. By 1969, there were 1,152 runners. In 1970, the number was limited to those who met a qualifying time.

Many runners feel that if they can complete a marathon they have passed the test. They may feel like dropping out during the run, and when they cross the finish line they might wonder why they were so crazy as to attempt it. Yet they know they have passed the test.

Jesus speaks of the storms of life that came to test a man. These trials of life prove whether a man is on solid rock or sinking sand. We do not desire nor seek out these trials, as a runner seeks out a good race. Yet when the trial is over, we know whether or not we have passed the test.

There are times when work is filled with problems, family life is filled with tensions, and our hearts are filled with doubts and questions. Then we are driven to cry out to God as David did, "Since I am afflicted and needy, let the Lord be mindful of me; Thou art my help and my deliverer; do not delay, O my God" (Ps. 40:17).

When you do this you will find, as David did, that God will

help and deliver you. Even though you are weak and tempted to give up, you will discover that with God's help you can pass the test. You can weather the storm. You can finish the race.

Do the trials you experience bring out the worst or the best in you?

How can you "build your house" on rock?

20. Beautiful Feet

How beautiful are the feet of those who bring good news (Rom. 10:15 NIV).

In the Scriptures, feet are referred to on many occasions. The most important feet are those of Jesus Christ. Nails were pounded through those feet and the lifeblood of the Savior poured out for all men. Because of His sinless life, His sacrificial death, and His powerful resurrection, God has exalted His Son to the highest place. "He [God] put all things in subjection under His feet, and gave Him as head over all things" (Eph. 1:22). Jesus is not only Savior but Lord. His nail-scarred feet are in authority over every person, problem, or power.

Jesus Christ has the most beautiful feet because He brought us the ultimate good news of our salvation. And Christians are also said to have beautiful feet when they follow in His footsteps and bring the Good News to others. When a Christian bears witness to Jesus, he is sharing the best news a person could ever hear. A witness is simply a person who tells what he has seen and knows to be true. We Christians know Jesus Christ is the Son of God, and we have seen Him change our lives.

Witnessing is so important that Paul tells us to have our feet fitted "with the preparation of the gospel of peace" (Eph. 6:15). Few runners begin their workout or run a race in a pair of leather dress shoes. In fact, just any old pair of tennis shoes won't do. They have to be just the right kind of shoes for protection, comfort, and speed.

Yet many Christians leave home without wearing their "gospel shoes." To put on gospel shoes is to maintain an attitude of alertness and readiness to share the Good News of

Jesus Christ wherever you go. It does not mean you witness to everyone you meet or "jam religion down their throats." It does mean that whenever an opportunity arises to speak for Christ, regardless of where you are, you take the opportunity.

To what extent have your feet been following in the footsteps of our Lord?

21. Handling Emotions

Be ready in season and out of season (2 Tim. 4:2).

We are all familiar with the phrase "the thrill of victory and the agony of defeat." Athletes experience a variety of emotions, such as loneliness, joy, pain, defeat, and exhilaration. Who could forget the picture of joy in Bruce Jenner's whole body after he crossed the finish line to win the Olympic decathlon title in 1976. As he ran that victory lap, waving his country's flag, thousands shared his joy.

But Paul urges us to keep on running the race even when we don't feel like it. "In season and out of season" we are to be in top spiritual shape, living with a sense of urgency and readiness. Many reach an emotional peak during some important event in their lives and then fall back into the doldrums afterward. Others experience life as a roller coaster of emotions, up one day and down the next, not understanding why.

The mature Christian is one who has learned to live life at a relatively steady pace. This sometimes involves ignoring our emotions. Feelings are a poor gauge of one's spiritual life. They change constantly and are affected by such simple things as the amount of sleep we get. No runner would drop out of a race just because he felt fear before the race started. He wouldn't use his feelings to determine his level of conditioning or his likelihood of doing well in the race. Rather he would ignore the fear and run anyway. Likewise, a Christian can ignore negative feelings that would paralyze him and do what must be done.

Christians base their lives not on their changeable emotions, but on their unchanging Savior. "Jesus Christ is the same yesterday and today, yes and forever" (Heb. 13:8). This means He is just as loving and powerful today as He was two thousand years ago when He healed the blind man. He will be just as wise and trustworthy tomorrow as He was at the beginning of time, when He created the universe. Christ is not affected by inflation, political turmoil, or changing styles and values. He is a solid rock upon which we can build our lives. As someone has said, "I may shake on the rock, but the rock never shakes under me."

Many people today are seeking some great experience that will transform their lives and put them on a constant emotional high. This is not only unrealistic but unbiblical. Jesus didn't promise to give us great feelings all the time. Rather, He promised to be with us through every situation (see Heb. 13:5). A. B. Simpson described this change of perspective in the hymn "Himself":

> Once it was the blessing,
> Now it is the Lord;
> Once it was the feeling,
> Now it is His Word;
> Once His gift I wanted,
> Now the Giver own;
> Once I sought for healing,
> Now Himself alone.

As we abandon the search for some great experience, or feeling, or spiritual gift, then we are set free to seek Christ Himself. We are liberated to live by the unchanging promises of God rather than by our own feelings. Some may ask, "Won't this make me an emotional blob?" Just the opposite! When Christ is the sole preoccupation of our lives, we find our joy in Him. This frees us from bondage to ourselves and we are able to "rejoice with those who rejoice, and weep with those who weep" (Rom. 12:15).

Emotions are fickle and will betray us. They have no power to permanently change or sustain our lives. But Christ and

His Word are reliable. They will never let us down. "Forever, O LORD, Thy word is settled in heaven. . . . If Thy law had not been my delight, then I would have perished in my affliction" (Ps. 119:89,92).

How have your emotions let you down in the past?

What unchanging promises of Christ can you base your life on today?

22. Bad Feet

There are . . . things the Lord hates . . . which are an
abomination to Him . . . feet that run rapidly to evil
(Prov. 6:16,18).

Dave Merrick looked like an upcoming Olympic hopeful for
the 1980s. He had so much talent and promise it seemed he
could not go wrong. But midway through his college career
he developed a foot-plant problem. Each time his foot landed
on the ground it transmitted a jarring shock to his knees. It
has been estimated that a person takes one thousand footsteps each mile. Dave ran about fifteen miles per day, which
means fifteen thousand hits to those bad feet each day. He cut
back to jogging, then walking, and finally experienced an end
to his promising running career. Bad feet and bone problems
killed his Olympic dreams.

Solomon's wisdom was respected by everyone in his day.
Today he still speaks through the Book of Proverbs. There he
directs our attention to feet that run quickly in the direction of
evil. In another place, Solomon says, "The ways of a man are
before the eyes of the LORD, and He watches all his paths. His
own iniquities will capture the wicked, and he will be held
with the cords of his sin" (Prov. 5:21,22). The word "paths"
means wagon tracks made by constant use. So this verse
refers to habits, things we do naturally and easily, because
we've done them that way a thousand times before.

Many runners develop a favorite course where they run
day after day. They don't have to think about which way to
go; it has become habitual through repetition. Some habits
are good such as running, or brushing your teeth, or saying
good morning to your wife. But a bad habit is very difficult to
change; a person can feel he is bound by unbreakable cords.

There is a way out. First, recognize that God sees and hates any evil habits we have fallen into. He is fully aware of the extent of the problem, and He has the power to break the cords that bind us. Second, confess and forsake the wrong path. Jesus said, "If your right hand makes you stumble, cut it off, and throw it from you" (Matt. 5:30). Forbid your hands or feet to go down those old, well-worn paths. Third, discover the good paths your feet should follow and begin running in the way of God's commands. Paul wrote, "Put on the Lord Jesus Christ, and make no provision for the flesh in regard to its lusts" (Rom. 13:14). This means, among other things, that I go only where Jesus would go, and do what He would do.

When a person begins to run in the right path, his feet will no longer be detestable to God but will be blessed by Him.

What wrong habits do you have?

What steps can you take to get on the right path?

23. Realizing Your Potential

Do not neglect the spiritual gift within you . . . (1 Tim. 4:14).

Author Jim Fixx reports that between 1977 and 1980 the number of runners in the United States increased from six million to twenty million. In 1982 it is estimated that more than forty million Americans are running. Some feel that this figure will eventually level off at about thirty million runners.

One of the reasons for the great popularity of running today is that it's a sport you can participate in regardless of your level of ability. Many of the "fun races" are filled with people who don't even care about their speed but are over-joyed that they just finished the race. Others are competing against themselves to improve their best time. Even men such as Frank Shorter and Bill Rodgers work at developing their potential as much as they work at winning races. This is a refreshing contrast to the win-at-all-costs competitiveness of our age.

The current popularity of running has drawn many into the sport who never did anything athletic before. Homemakers are running beside busy executives. People in wheelchairs are developing athletic potential they never knew they had. Children run in races alongside their grandparents. Realizing hidden potential is a beautiful thing.

When a person becomes a Christian he receives the gift of the Holy Spirit, who comes to live inside him (see Acts 2:38). At this time he also receives one or more spiritual gifts which he is to exercise for the building up of fellow Christians (see Rom. 12:6–8). One may have a gift of serving while another has a gift of encouraging. Some people have many gifts, while others have only a few. The important thing is not how gifted

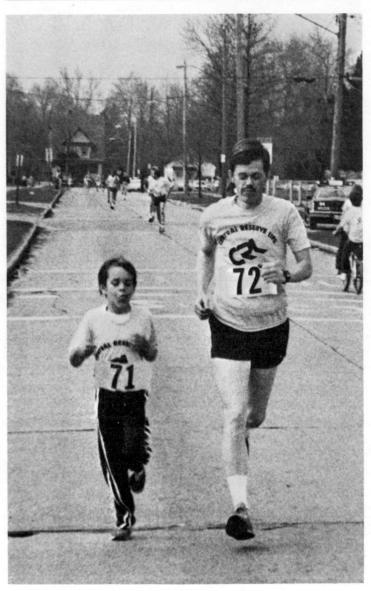

a person is, but how faithful he is to humbly use his gifts for building others up. Many Christians neglect their gifts and live narrow, selfish lives.

Timothy was a shy young fellow who easily withdrew from responsibility and people. Paul had to remind him to "kindle afresh the gift of God which is in you" (2 Tim. 1:6). Timothy easily could have let that flame burn low until it was just a dimly burning wick. There are too many timid Timothys today living far below their potential.

Paul went on to say to Timothy: "For God has not given us a spirit of timidity, but of power and love and discipline" (2 Tim. 1:7). Perhaps some will say, "But I could never be a victorious, outgoing Christian. I'm too shy; it's not my personality." The issue is not one of personality but of character. God is able to give boldness and courage even to a shy, quiet person. Courage does not mean running about as a raving extrovert. Simply, courage means doing what should be done and what God commands to be done. Developing and using your gifts is an act of love toward others. The one who does this in God's strength is the one who will live up to his potential.

Success is not what we have achieved compared to someone else, but what we have achieved compared to the abilities God has given us.

In what areas are you failing to live up to your potential?

How can claiming the promise of 2 Timothy 1:7 bring you victory over shyness and fear?

24. The Fastest Disciple

Peter therefore went forth, and the other disciple, and they were going to the tomb. And the two were running together; and the other disciple ran ahead faster than Peter, and came to the tomb first; and stooping and looking in, he saw the linen wrappings lying there; but he did not go in. Simon Peter therefore also came, following him, and entered the tomb; and he beheld the linen wrappings lying there, and the face-cloth, which had been on His head, not lying with the linen wrappings, but rolled up in a place by itself. So the other disciple who had first come to the tomb entered then also, and he saw and believed (John 20:3–8).

In this account we find that John outran Peter to the tomb. These discouraged and defeated men suddenly had something worth running for. Although John had the greater speed, both men made the same discovery—the tomb was empty and Jesus was alive!

We could go to Israel today and make that same run to the empty tomb that the two disciples made. But far more exciting than retracing those steps is knowing the presence of the risen Christ in our hearts through His Holy Spirit. Jesus said, "It is to your advantage that I go away; for if I do not go away, the Helper shall not come to you; but if I go, I will send Him to you" (John 16:7).

The living Christ is still at work on earth doing miracles and teaching people. But today He is not limited by His physical body; He works through His Holy Spirit. We may not be one of the fastest runners, but we can glory in the risen Christ just as Peter and John did.

What evidence is there in your life that the resurrected Christ is at work in you through His Spirit?

25. Teamwork

. . . from [Christ] the whole body, being fitted and held together by that which every joint supplies, according to the proper working of each individual part, causes the growth of the body for the building up of itself in love (Eph. 4:16).

There are many team sports—baseball, football, basketball, to name a few. Running is one sport that requires very little teamwork except in the case of a relay race, when precision timing and coordination are required as two runners exchange a baton.

But within the body of each runner there is an unbelievable amount of teamwork. The brain sends out signals that are obeyed by thousands of nerves and muscles. The skin and glands respond. The heart, lungs, and blood vessels all become deeply involved and magnificently coordinated with the other functions of the body—all to produce the simple movement we call "running." Surely we are "fearfully and wonderfully made"! (Ps. 139:14).

It is this magnificent coordination and interdependence within the human body that Paul uses to illustrate how individual Christians should relate to the church as a whole. Each person has a different function (see 1 Cor. 12). One may be like the eye, another like a hand or a foot. Each part is important to the whole.

Although there are some blind runners today, it is very difficult to run without the use of your eyes. On the other hand, even if you had a good set of eyes, if your legs didn't work you wouldn't be a runner. So each Christian has a different function within the body of Christ. The church cannot run smoothly unless each person does his part.

A sense of inferiority keeps many people from doing their part in the body of Christ. "If the ear should say, 'Because I am not an eye, I am not a part of the body,' it is not for this reason any the less a part of the body. If the whole body were an eye, where would the hearing be?" (1 Cor. 12:16,17).

Suppose, at the beginning of a race, a six-foot eyeball rolled up to the starting line. It could probably see the whole course at a glance, but it would never hear the gun go off. And besides, no Nikes have been made to fit something of that shape! To have a complete body all the parts are essential.

Your gift or function may not seem very important. You may feel you're more like a lowly foot than the beautiful eyes that get all the attention. But ask any runner how important his foot or even one toe is to him.

Every Christian must exercise his gift in order for Christ's body to function effectively and bring glory to God.

Do you know what your role is in the body of Christ?

How can your overcoming inferiority help the whole church?

26. Strict Training

Do you not know that in a race all the runners run, but only one gets the prize? Run in such a way as to get the prize. Everyone who competes in the games goes into strict training. They do it to get a crown of laurel that will not last, but we do it to get a crown that will last forever. Therefore, I do not run like a man running aimlessly; I do not fight like a man shadow boxing. No, I beat my body and make it my slave so that after I have preached to others, I myself will not be disqualified for the prize (1 Cor. 9:24–27 NIV).

The recipients of this letter at Corinth could readily understand Paul's athletic illustration. Each year Corinth hosted the Isthmian games, second only to the Olympic games. Everyone had watched the athletes sweat and work to win the coveted crown of laurel leaves. Paul points out that this crown will not last. Even a modern gold medal will eventually lose its initial significance. But the Christian competes for a crown that will endure through all time and eternity. How much more should a believer in Christ go into strict spiritual training to receive the eternal prize of heavenly rewards!

Frank Shorter, who won a gold medal in the marathon at the 1972 Olympics, said he was no different from anyone else on the street. If he would stop practicing for three months, he would be the same as any other jogger. The same is true in the spiritual life.

One of the most important disciplines for a Christian to practice is a daily "quiet time." Many have testified that this brief time of meeting with God each morning for fifteen to thirty minutes has revolutionized their lives. It is a discipline one chooses to practice, much like running. It should be done regardless of feelings. A person who studies the Bible fifteen

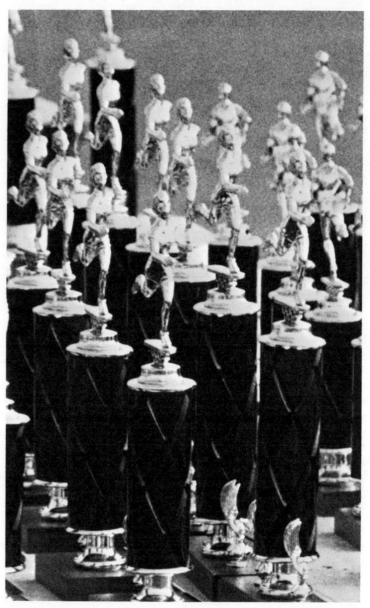

minutes a day for ten years will have logged 912 hours of direct Bible study! That is more than the hours in four years of Bible school!

Each time spiritual disciplines are practiced, spiritual muscles develop. When they are ignored, spiritual muscles atrophy, leaving a person weak and useless in the most important area of life. Dr. Kenneth Cooper, author of *Aerobics* and a dedicated Christian, has said, "If you want to improve your physical fitness, you have to exercise daily. If you want to improve your spiritual fitness, there is no way you can read your Bible once a week and expect to improve. You have to set goals" (*Worldwide Challenge*, March, 1979).

Frank Shorter was swept into stardom by his performance in the 1972 Olympics. Many consider that race the beginning of the modern running boom. Frank took second place in the marathon at the 1976 Olympics, but then his performances began to deteriorate. It was discovered that he had been running on a severely injured left foot, and surgery was required.

Today he is past the height of his running career, yet he still runs one hundred miles a week, primarily because he loves to run. Clearly, this is a man dedicated to "strict training." In a recent interview, he reflected on his school days, when many people got satisfaction from doing less than other people were doing. Frank said, "I'm just the opposite. I'd rather outwork my opposition."

If a man can be this dedicated to training himself physically, how much more should a Christian dedicate himself to Jesus Christ. His disciples must be characterized by daily spiritual disciplines. The Lord and Creator of the universe deserves nothing less.

Are you more dedicated to physical fitness than you are to spiritual fitness?

What disciplines should you be building into your spiritual training program?

27. Uniforms

Clothe yourselves with the Lord Jesus Christ (Rom. 13:14 NIV).

All athletes are concerned about their uniforms. For football or hockey, the uniform is essential for safety. Even runners are concerned about their uniforms. There are sweat suits that not only keep runners at the right temperature but also reflect light to protect them at night. Some of the better running shoes are now priced near one hundred dollars. Shorts and shirts must be lightweight. A good watch is also an important part of a runner's equipment.

The Bible makes a number of references to uniforms worn by Christians. In our relationship to God we are clothed with the garments of salvation and robes of righteousness (see Is. 61:10).

In our relationship to each other we are to have the clothing of godly virtues. "Clothe yourselves with compassion, kindness, humility, gentleness and patience. . . . And over all these virtues put on love" (Col. 3:12,14 NIV). The fact that we are to put these virtues on like clothes demonstrates that love is something we do, not something we feel.

A Christian also needs to wear a particular uniform in his relationship to the enemy, Satan. "Put on the full armor of God, that you may be able to stand firm against the schemes of the devil" (Eph. 6:11). We live in enemy-occupied territory, Paul stressed, and to live successfully and win battles we must wear the belt of truth, the helmet of salvation, and the other parts of armor listed in Ephesians 6:14–18. The goal is to be strong and stand firm against Satan's attack.

The primary uniform a Christian is to wear is Jesus Christ Himself! We are told to put Him on, to clothe ourselves with

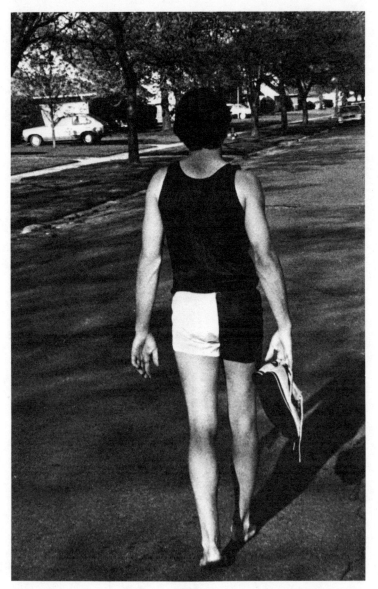

Him. We belong to Him and are named after Him, and when people look at us they should see Him. Therefore, we need to have His eyes to see things as He sees them, His feet to go where He would go, His hands to do His work, His mind to think His thoughts, and His heart to feel His concerns.

The fact is that only Jesus Christ can live the Christian life. He will live it through us if we allow Him to. Attempting to live up to the high standards of the Bible in this dark world would be like a 120-pound weakling trying to play fullback without a uniform against the Pittsburgh Steelers. But even the weakest person who puts on the Lord Jesus Christ will be able to "be strong in the Lord, and in the strength of His might" (Eph. 6:10).

Read Ephesians 6:10–18. Why does Paul emphasize the need for the "full" armor of God?

What parts of the spiritual uniform do you need to begin wearing?

28. The Man Who Ran the Wrong Way

But Jonah ran away from the LORD and headed for Tarshish. He went down to Joppa, where he found a ship bound for that port. After paying the fare, he went aboard and sailed for Tarshish to flee from the LORD (Jon. 1:3 NIV).

Jonah's jog was not just a run to the sea coast for the exercise. He was trying to escape from the mission God had given him. He did not want to go to Nineveh and preach to the people, because they were enemies of the Jews. Jonah would rather have seen them judged and destroyed by God than for them to repent and be saved. So he began to run in the opposite direction of Nineveh. But God apprehended Jonah in his flight and gave him a free trip to Nineveh (in a fish). The record is plain: Man cannot run away from God's will without paying the price.

Like Jonah, many people today are running. They are running away from their marriages, from difficult circumstances, and from the "boredom" of the straight life. In reality, they are trying to run away from God and His perfect will. They think that doing God's will makes a person miserable and that only their own plans will bring happiness.

But the opposite is true. "'I know the plans that I have for you,' declares the LORD, 'plans for welfare and not for calamity, to give you a future and a hope'" (Jer. 29:11). God pursued and apprehended Jonah, not to punish him but to bless and use him.

Have you been trying to run away from God's perfect will for your life?

What must you do to begin running in God's way again?

29. The Pain of Endurance

Jesus . . . who for the joy set before Him endured the cross, despising the shame, and has sat down at the right hand of the throne of God (Heb. 12:2).

Grete Waitz, who has run the second fastest marathon of any woman in the world as of November 1981, expressed her philosophy of training: "If you want to develop as a runner you have to do some painful training." In a few words, her philosophy is "no pain, no gain." Most successful runners would agree.

Today people want instant success. They want to advance and progress without any accompanying pain or discomfort. "No sweat" is the byword of many. Francis Schaeffer says the goal of modern man focuses on two values: personal peace and affluence. Man wants nothing to disturb his happiness, his wealth, or his ever-increasing pleasure.

God calls us to holiness more than He does to happiness. Happiness is a natural by-product of holiness. Pursuing personal holiness or God-likeness will involve some difficulties and pain, but the Bible exhorts us to make any sacrifice in order to reach our goal of holy living. You have not yet resisted to the point of shedding blood in your striving against sin (Heb. 12:4). The point is we should be willing to go to any length—even death—to avoid sinning.

Some Christians feel there is something wrong if they are not happy every minute of every day. Yet Jesus was not always happy. He didn't enjoy fasting and being tempted by the devil. He didn't enjoy being misunderstood by His family and rejected by the religious leaders. He didn't enjoy being in anguish in the Garden of Gethsemane. He didn't enjoy carrying his cross to Calvary and having the nails driven through His hands and feet. Yet "for the joy set before Him [He] endured the cross" (Heb. 12:2).

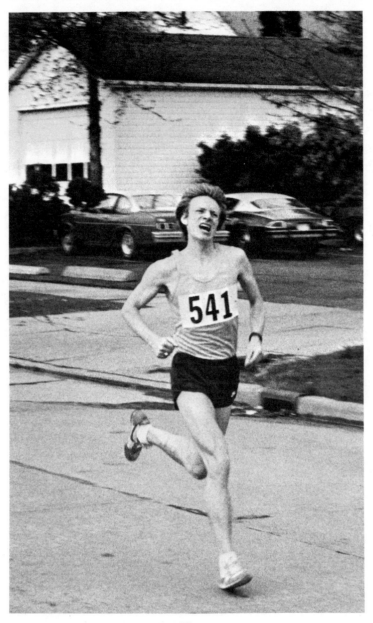

Jesus Christ was called the "Holy One of God" (John 6:69). Even though He was a completely sinless and holy man, He suffered a great deal of pain. Yet He was the most joyful man who ever lived. Speaking of Christ, the Scriptures say, "Thou hast loved righteousness and hated lawlessness; therefore God, Thy God, hath anointed Thee with the oil of gladness above Thy companions" (Heb. 1:9). There was a cause-and-effect relationship between His holiness and His joy. One led to the other.

Just as a successful marathon runner is willing to pay the price of 100 to 120 miles of painful training each week, so a Christian must be willing to pay the price of suffering to experience the joy of victorious Christian living. What kind of suffering? It may be in the form of rejection because of our morals or our witness (see Matt 5:10–12). It may be the weariness of doing good (see Gal. 6:9), or having to endure a situation that seems endless (see Ps. 40:1,2), or perhaps being misunderstood by one's family (see Mark 3:20,21).

Peter exhorts us to keep this suffering in perspective. "In this you greatly rejoice, even though now for a little while, if necessary, you have been distressed by various trials" (1 Pet. 1:6). At the time, painful trials seem like they are lasting forever. But in reality, and with eternity in view, they last only "a little while." Peter urges us to remember that painful experiences are like the fire that refines gold.

All of us experience pain, frustration, disappointment, and stress. As we set our minds on the fact that these problems will help to refine and purify our faith, we will know the peace that passes and transcends all logical understanding (see Phil. 4:7).

Can you think of painful experiences of your past that have proved good for you?

What suffering are you now experiencing in which you can claim Romans 8:28?

30. Disqualified

I buffet my body and make it my slave, lest possibly, after I have preached to others, I myself should be disqualified (1 Cor. 9:27).

Big Ben Plucknett was a powerful man who felt driven to set a world record in the discus throw. He spent thousands of hours in training. But in 1981, he became unhappy with his progress, seeing little improvement even with increased work. He began using anabolic steroids, which accelerated his muscle development. Big Ben did improve—so much so that he set a new world record. After the competition the athletes were tested for drugs and when traces of the steroids were found in his blood, Ben's world record was stripped from him and he was disqualified and banned from future competition. He broke the rules and suffered the shame of disqualification.

As confident and positive as the apostle Paul was, he seemed to be haunted by the fear that he might be disqualified from the race. And as everyone knows, there can be no possibility of reward for a disqualified runner. What temptations could put such fear and concern into the great apostle?

Paul was concerned about the physical drives of his body. He was concerned that he might preach a message on self-control and then live in self-indulgence. Others before had experienced similar tragedies. Eli the priest had given in to the hunger drive and died a fat, self-indulgent old man (see 1 Sam. 1–4). King David had given in to his sex drive and brought misery upon his family and his nation (see 2 Sam. 11ff.). Paul did not want to make similar mistakes.

Paul chose the course of self-denial, forcing his body to be his slave, not his master. Every athlete knows what it means to command his body. At six o'clock, before breakfast, my body rarely desires to go running. But my mind commands it to do so, and it meekly obeys in willing submission. Every runner practices keeping his body in a position of slavery to his mind.

The same principles that lead to success in the athletic realm will produce prosperity in the moral and spiritual realm. The world's slogan is "indulge yourself," but Jesus taught, "Deny yourself."

Why is the fear of disqualification a healthy fear?

In what areas do you need to begin ruling your physical drives?

31. Listen to the Coach

The sheep listen to his voice (John 10:3 NIV).

The track coach in my high school produced many excellent distance runners. Each day he would prescribe a difficult workout schedule for us to follow. All the distance runners were very dedicated to the coach—until one spring when a stranger began hanging around the track at workout times. He was an older man, and he seemed to know all about distance running. So the milers began following his advice and doing his workout schedule.

As we prepared for the first meet, our coach quietly observed us following the stranger's advice. We had won the state championship in cross country that fall, so we were expected to win the first invitational relays of the outdoor track season as well. Instead, we placed a disappointing tenth.

The following Monday, we all listened to the coach's workout plan and followed it carefully. We knew that in following the stranger we had been listening to the wrong voice.

Jesus claimed to be the Good Shepherd (see John 10:11). Those who are truly His sheep will hear and obey His voice. Many other competing voices seek to distract us. Satan is the wolf who wants to scatter the sheep. He can disguise himself so that people think they are listening to the right voice. But in reality, he is the thief who "comes only to steal, and kill, and destroy" (see John 10:10). He is the stranger who promises much but delivers little.

One of Satan's primary attacks upon believers is to accuse them (see Rev. 12:10). He does this by planting thoughts in our minds that focus upon all our failures and defeats. His basic message to us is, "You're no good! You're no good!

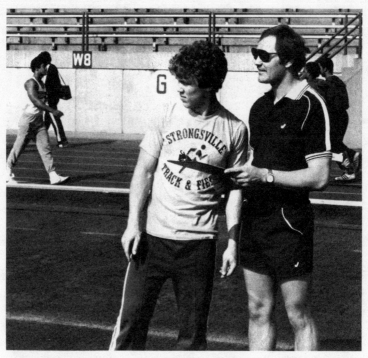

You're no good!" So we are tricked by this voice into believing a lie.

All the while, Jesus Christ whispers to us, "Do not fear, for I have redeemed you; I have called you by name; you are Mine! . . . you are precious in My sight . . . since I love you" (Is. 43:1,4). This is the voice of the Good Shepherd, which we must recognize and heed. He knows we are sinners, but He has shed His blood to forgive those sins and now He sees us as forgiven. If this is how God sees us, then so must we see ourselves. Reject the voice of the stranger and listen to the voice of your Friend and Shepherd.

In what areas might you be listening to the wrong voices?

How can you better listen for the voice of Christ?

32. The Aimless Runner

I run in such a way, as not without aim. (1 Cor. 9:26).

The apostle Paul saw himself as a runner and his whole life and ministry as a great race. His goal was to develop such an intimate, personal relationship with Jesus that he would become fully like Him in character and conduct. "One thing I do: forgetting what lies behind and reaching forward to what lies ahead, I press on toward the goal for the prize of the upward call of God in Christ Jesus" (Phil. 3:13,14). Paul pictures a runner straining with every ounce of energy toward the finish line, leaning with outstretched arms toward the tape.

How different this is from the aimless kind of living most people pursue today, toying with one trivial activity after another. Paul's life was not characterized by aimlessness. He didn't say, "These fifteen things I do. . ." but "this one thing I do"! Rather than drifting through life, he pressed hard toward a goal.

In the Pan-American games in Mexico City, a boy commented to a sports writer, "With God's help, I'm going to set a new world's record this year." No one paid much attention to him. But when Lou Jones approached the starting line for the 400-meter dash, he was determined to reach his goal. Going around the curve, Lou and two other runners were only inches apart. Spectators could see the effects of the high altitude on the runners as the men gasped for air. Pumping and driving that last twenty yards, Lou dove for the tape, snapping it not more than an inch in front of the others as he collapsed unconscious on the track. After receiving oxygen and being revived, Lou learned that he had set a new world record of 45.4 seconds. Lou Jones pursued a goal with all his energy.

Many today have lost sight of any dominant goal for their lives. They are torn this way and that by hundreds of pressures and competing priorities. Some pursue fame, while others seek pleasure, or money, or "self-fulfillment." Thousands give themselves so totally to their jobs that Christlike character and family life suffer.

God is honored by people who, like Paul, choose the right life goal and then pour all their energy into fulfilling it, considering all other successes secondary to knowing Christ and becoming like Him.

Only the person who makes Jesus Christ his first priority will be truly satisfied (see Matt. 6:33). This may cause him to be out of step with the world, but he'll be in step with God's plan because he is fulfilling the reason for which he was created.

Forsake aimless living. Press toward the goal!

To what extent is your life dominated by one great goal?

How would a single-minded pursuit of Christlikeness improve your personal life, family life, work life, and social life?

33. Repetition

Rejoice in the Lord always; again I will say, rejoice!
(Phil. 4:4).

Doing something over and over again is the basis of all physical training. The whole concept of a daily workout is based on repetition. A second baseman works on the double play until it becomes second nature to him. A tennis player practices his serve for endless hours. Weightlifters repeat a particular lift or press. Many track runners practice "repetition training" when they run at a high speed, wait for a full recovery, then run again, repeating the process over and over.

Repetition is just as important in the spiritual life. There are many activities we are instructed to do again and again, such as taking the Lord's Supper, fellowshipping with other Christians, and reading the Bible. One of the most important spiritual activities we are to repeat is the practice of rejoicing. Paul stressed it over and over again in the Philippian Letter, even mentioning it twice in one verse (Phil. 4:4).

We wonder how this practice can be maintained when the times seem so dark and the problems surrounding us so numerous. But Paul did not say we should rejoice because of our circumstances or just when things are going well. That would leave many people little opportunity for rejoicing. Rather, we are to rejoice "in the Lord," who never changes and is always worthy of our praise. Just as a dedicated runner ignores the weather conditions and works out anyway, so a committed Christian ignores his circumstances and rejoices in Christ, regardless of the situation.

Paul practiced what he preached when he was put in prison at Philippi. He and Silas were stripped, beaten, and flogged before being thrown into prison, but the Bible says that at midnight they were praying and singing hymns to God (see Acts 16:25). They didn't look at their negative circumstances but praised their unchanging God, who brought them joy in a very dark hour.

We live in an age of scoffing, grumbling, and negativism. Only the strong medicine of thanksgiving, praise, and rejoicing will keep us from being infected. But we need to take this medicine daily, hourly, even moment by moment. "Rejoice always . . . for this is God's will for you in Christ Jesus" (1 Thess. 5:16–18).

Rejoicing is a response we choose, just as we choose to grumble or complain. The runner who repeats his workout over and over will eventually reap the benefits. The Christian who rejoices constantly will reap the spiritual rewards of this conditioning. "All the days of the afflicted are bad, but a cheerful heart has a continual feast (Prov. 15:15).

How many times did you rejoice today? Compare this to the number of times you grumbled.

What attributes of Jesus Christ can you rejoice in when your circumstances are dark?

34. Run for Your Life

And though she [Potiphar's wife] spoke to Joseph day after day, he refused to go to bed with her or even be with her. One day he went into the house to attend to his duties, and none of the household servants was inside. She caught him by his cloak and said, "Come to bed with me!" But he left his cloak in her hand and ran out of the house (Gen. 39:10–12 NIV).

This short sprint was one of the greatest runs of all time. Joseph left his cloak but won the trophy for purity and self-control. As manager of Potiphar's household, he knew that everything was entrusted to him except Potiphar's wife. So he kept his distance from this flirtatious woman. He must have known the truth of Proverbs 7:27 and 5:8: "Her house is the way to Sheol, descending to the chambers of death. . . . Keep your way far from her." When she tried to seduce him, Joseph took off running.

With some temptations, the correct strategy is to stand your ground and resist the tempter. But in the case of temptations to lust, the strategy is always to run away as fast as you can. Joseph is an Old Testament illustration of a New Testament truth. Paul wrote, "Flee from youthful lusts, and pursue righteousness, faith, love and peace, with those who call on the Lord from a pure heart" (2 Tim. 2:22).

To stay and try to resist will likely end in defeat. Sprinters must get a good start, and Joseph knew that if he delayed his dash to find out how strong he was, he would only discover how weak he was. So he ran, right away and quickly.

Joseph shows us two wonderful paradoxes. In recognizing his weakness, he became strong. And running away, he showed moral courage, thereby protecting his purity and the honor of God's name.

Do you run quickly from lustful temptations, or do you delay your dash and become ensnared?

How can you practically apply this truth to situations where you are tempted?

35. The Second Wind

He breathed on them, and said to them, "Receive the Holy Spirit" (John 20:22).

A common experience of runners is to come to a point of exhaustion during a race and then to find some deep reserves within themselves, enabling them to continue with new and fresh energy.

Many Christians are at the point of exhaustion. They have used up all their resources, and weariness is about to overtake them. They are tired of trying and weary of defeat. They are discouraged with themselves and disillusioned with others. It's at this point that God says, "Good! I've been waiting for you to get to this place. Now that you've learned how hopeless it is to depend upon your own energy, you are ready to learn what it is like to depend upon My inexhaustible supply."

God is often considered a last resort. We try everything before we let God show us what He can do. Through all the self-effort, we learn valuable lessons about not trusting in ourselves. We also learn to go to God first and seek His help immediately. David said, "Unless the LORD builds the house, they labor in vain who build it" (Ps. 127:1). Jesus said, "Apart from Me you can do nothing" (John 15:5). All the efforts we expend apart from Christ are empty and worthless, accomplishing nothing of real value.

Jesus' disciples were miserable failures while He was on earth. They got into petty arguments about who was the greatest; they fell asleep in prayer meetings; Peter, their spokesman, frequently put his foot in his mouth. Jesus taught about the necessity of His upcoming death and His resurrection after three days. But the disciples tried to keep Him from the cross, and they didn't believe in His resurrection until it was proved to them. At His trial, they all forsook Him.

But then they found the second wind, and that turned them into shining successes, boldly preaching for Christ and winning people to Him. The first wind was their own wisdom and power. The second wind came when they received the Holy Spirit and began to plug into His wisdom and power. When Jesus gave the gift of the Spirit to His followers, the very breath of God came into them. Paul prayed that we might come to know "the surpassing greatness of His power toward us who believe" (Eph. 1:19) and that we "may be filled up to all the fulness of God" (Eph. 3:19).

Dr. Albert B. Simpson was a preacher in the late 1800s. He suffered from many infirmities and disabilities, and he lived with continual discouragement. It took him until Wednesday to get over the exhausting effects of his Sunday sermon. One weekend, on a retreat, he heard a chorus being sung: "My Jesus is Lord of Lords: No man can work like Him." The thought deeply affected him, and he took Christ to be his Lord and to work for him.

After the new work of the Spirit in Dr. Simpson's life, he worked and labored for years with great ease.

> The first three years after I was healed I preached more than a thousand sermons, and held sometimes more than twenty meetings in one week. I do not remember once feeling exhausted from a single service all that time. . . . He called me into a special work involving fourfold more labor than any previous period in my life. . . . It has been a continual delight and seldom any burden or fatigue, and much, very much easier in every way than the far lighter tasks of former years.[1]

This is the second wind: to be filled with the Holy Spirit so that all your energy and effort are coming from an outside

---

[1]A. E. Thompson, *A. B. Simpson: His Life and Work* (Harrisburg, PA: Christian Publications, 1960).

source. When the breath of God fills your lungs, You can run without growing weary.

At this point in your life, would you consider yourself filled with the Holy Spirit?

What steps can you take to experience this new power? See Acts 5:32.

36. Hitting the Wall

Then Jezebel sent a messenger to Elijah, saying, "So may the gods do to me and even more, if I do not make your life as the life of one of them by tomorrow about this time." And he was afraid and ran for his life.... [he] sat down under a juniper tree; and he requested for himself that he might die, and said, "It is enough; now, O LORD, take my life, for I am not better than my fathers." And he lay down and slept under a juniper tree; and behold, there was an angel touching him, and he said to him, "Arise, eat" (1 Kin. 19:2–5).

A marathon is twenty-six miles long. While making this run, some very capable runners have experienced what they call "hitting the wall"—a feeling of impending collapse at about the twenty-mile mark, due to a physical and emotional drain on their systems. It is as if their bodies are shouting to them, "Quit; it's not worth it. Just step off the course!" Some very capable men of God have experienced a similar phenomenon in their spiritual lives.

Elijah was one of the greatest prophets of all time. He had just confronted the prophets of Baal, boldly and successfully. Then Jezebel threatened his life, and the courageous prophet turned into a defeated and fearful runner. The spirit of bold confrontation had left him, and he ran to save his own skin. He sat under a tree, defeated and despairing of life itself. Elijah had given up and dropped out of the race.

Elijah's experience illustrates a New Testament truth: "Let him who thinks he stands take heed lest he fall" (1 Cor. 10: 12). A high is often followed by a low. Elijah's depression also illustrates the close relationship among the spirit, soul, and body. His physical and emotional exhaustion led to spiritual depression. God's prescription for him was simply to rest and have a good meal.

A depressed person never thinks clearly. At first, Elijah was afraid he might die. Then, after he escaped, he prayed that he would die. The apostle Paul affirmed the wonderful confidence of the Christian when he wrote, "For to me, to live is Christ, and to die is gain" (Phil. 1:21). Paul, like Elijah, was threatened with death many times. But he didn't fear death, because he knew that to be in heaven and see Christ face to face would be truly glorious. So a Christian need not fear death.

When Elijah prayed for his own death, he was in the dungeon of despair. Paul again shows us the right attitude: "For to me, to live is Christ." Even in the most difficult circumstances, knowing the Lord Jesus and His power at work within us makes life worth living. The Christian need not run away from difficult circumstances, but rather look expectantly to Jesus to see what He will do. He is an ever present help in time of trouble.

What situations have brought fear or despair into your life?

How can you avoid Elijah's mistakes?

37. Weekend Athletes

Prove yourself doers of the word, and not merely hearers who delude themselves (James 1:22).

Each of us knows at least one weekend athlete. He enjoyed sports in his high-school days and maybe even in college. Now he's in his mid-thirties and about fifteen pounds overweight, with a bulge in his midsection and a great love for food. He also has a busy schedule and lots of pressure and stress in his job. But he still has the competitive urges from his school days, so about once a month he goes out on the tennis or basketball court and madly overdoes it for two hours. Some label him the "Type A" personality—the kind most prone to heart attacks. He practices a dangerous form of exercise.

There is a spiritual weekend athlete of the same type. Some call him the "Sunday-only Christian." He prays, listens to the Bible, and appears to be spiritual—one day each week. The rest of the week he engages in no spiritual exercise; in fact, he practices considerable self-indulgence. It's a dangerous place to be spiritually.

The man who learns God's will intellectually but never acts upon it or applies it to his life is a spiritual weakling. He is like a man who subscribes to all the runners' magazines, watches track meets on TV, attends local marathons as a spectator, and cheers enthusiastically—but never runs even once around the block. He is knowledgeable and even supportive, but he gains no personal benefits from the sport. He could quote the world-record time for the mile, but he couldn't run a mile if his life depended on it.

Jesus said that the storms of life will eventually test the spiritual weakling and reveal that his house was built on sand. He listened respectfully to Christ's Word, but he never acted upon it. The man whose house is built on rock is the one who listens to and obeys Christ's word, putting it into practice seven days out of seven (Matt. 7:24–27). This man will pass the test. He's no weekend athlete.

Muscles must be used often and regularly if they are to be kept in shape. Obedience is the exercise that develops spiritual muscles. Every day we should study the Bible and ask, "Lord, what would you have me do or be today?" It's amazing how each day God will reveal His specific will to us. It may be an attitude we should have, a practice we should avoid, or a job we should do. As we obey His will daily, our spiritual muscles will become stronger.

Prayer is another form of spiritual exercise. Praying once a week is worse than not praying at all. It deceives one into thinking he is really a praying person. In reality, he is relating to God from a distance, and few of his prayers will be answered. David's attitude was quite different. "In the morning, O LORD, Thou wilt hear my voice; in the morning I will order my prayer to Thee and eagerly watch" (Ps. 5:3). The person who practices daily, believing prayer will see God answer and will become spiritually strong as a result.

Muscles can only be developed by using them, and prayer and obedience are two ways to exercise spiritual muscles.

How can you begin a program to develop spiritual muscles?

What commands of Christ do you need to begin obeying today?

38. Run and Kiss

Then Esau ran to meet him and embraced him and fell on his neck and kissed him, and they wept (Gen. 33:4).

When Jacob saw Esau approaching with four hundred men, he must have been overcome with guilt and fear. Years earlier he had cheated Esau out of his birthright. Now the day of reckoning had come; surely he would experience the vengeance of a bitter brother. When they were close enough to see each other clearly, Esau ran toward Jacob. What was his intention? Did he have a knife concealed under his coat? Much to Jacob's surprise and relief, he was embraced and forgiven by his brother. Esau demonstrated one of the greatest virtues—forgiveness.

Forgiveness is so important that we should run to give it. The meaning of Esau's kiss is that now nothing stood between himself and Jacob. All had been put behind them, even as God has put our sins behind Him and forgotten them.

Another Old Testament figure who forgave his brothers was Joseph. After they sold him into slavery, he rose to power in Egypt. Years later, when he saved their lives and revealed himself to them, Joseph embraced and kissed his brothers. He relieved their guilt with his radiant confidence in God's purpose and power to work all things for good. "You meant evil against me, but God meant it for good in order to bring about this present result, to preserve many people alive" (Gen. 50:20).

It is impossible for any of us to make it through life without being hurt and wounded by someone. We can run away from them in bitterness, saying, "I'll never forgive them as long as I live," and destroy ourselves in the process. Or we can run toward them when we see them moving toward us and offer forgiveness. Even when the one who offended us never ac-knowledges any wrongdoing, we can still take the initiative in our own hearts to exercise Jesus Christ's attitude: "Father, forgive them; for they do not know what they are doing" (Luke 23:34).

Make a list of people you've never forgiven for something they've done to you. Use Jesus' words to specifically forgive each one in prayer.

Make a list of any people you need to ask forgiveness of. Begin with the first one on the list.

39. The Joy of Running

*. . . like a champion rejoicing to run his course (Ps. 19:5
NIV).*

Non-runners never can understand the enjoyment a runner finds out on those roads. To the uninvolved it seems like
sheer nonsense. Why would people go out there day after
day, rain or shine, putting their bodies through such grueling
torture? Running has been described in such glowing and
poetic terms ("Leaping through space as the gently falling
leaves greeted me with joy") that one tends to disbelieve that
it's really all that great.

I suppose the same is true of the unbeliever listening to a
Christian's testimony. It sounds all too good to be true. He
knows enough of Christ's teaching to realize that the Christian life is one of self-denial and discipline. How can that lead
to joy?

Of course, the spectator will never know the joys of running until he commits himself to participation. Then the discipline and sweat that he used to scorn become the very things
that lead to a new freedom—not a freedom to avoid sweat,
exertion, and discipline, but a freedom to practice it. The
spectator is not even free to run for a bus without feeling
exhausted. The runner has gained a new freedom of health
and energy that leads to joy and life on a higher plane.

It's the same in the Christian life. Paul says, "It was for
freedom that Christ set us free" (Gal. 5:1). This is not a
freedom to disobey God and indulge ourselves. Rather,
through the indwelling Spirit, Christ sets us free from bondage to ourselves so that we can choose to obey Him. We no
longer have to be enslaved to our sinful natures (Rom. 6:6).

Therefore, what looks like a negative life to the unbeliever is in reality a joyful liberation to live the life we were meant to live. The Christian can say, along with David, "I have rejoiced in the way of Thy testimonies, as much as in all riches" (Ps. 119:14).

To what extent are you experiencing joy in your Christian life?

Praise Him for the freedom you have received.

40. Walk—Don't Run

Anyone who runs ahead and does not continue in the teachings of Christ does not have God (2 John 9 NIV).

We have all seen those funny-looking people on TV who walk as fast as they can. As they bob along with their arms cocked and their heads wagging, it looks like they will break into a trot at any moment. Yet with great self-control, they refrain from running. For them, running would mean disqualification from the race.

There is a spiritual lesson to be learned from these disciplined athletes. John, in his brief second letter, warns of the dangers of false teachers and antichrists, those who would deceive Christians into following a doctrine different from the teachings of Jesus Christ. Anyone who involves himself in a cult like this has run ahead of his Lord and is no longer following Christ. He is like a walker who broke the rules and ran, disqualifying himself from the race.

To "run ahead" would be to begin believing truths that were not taught by Christ, to add to His teaching, or to twist or distort the Bible—to go beyond the boundary lines set down by the writers of Scripture.

Christians should never run ahead of Christ but always follow Him. The standard of Christian teaching has always been the Lord Jesus Christ—God incarnate dying for our sins, rising from the dead, and ascending into heaven to be seated at the right hand of the Father. We live in an age when more and more people are rejecting these basic truths. Never before have there sprung up more cults and sects that deceive people and lead them astray.

The true Christian is to be characterized by walking closely behind Christ. John says we are to walk in the truth (v. 4), to walk in obedience (v. 6), and to walk in love (v. 6). In order to walk in the truth, we must reject error and embrace Scripture. In the last days many will seek to deceive God's people; believers must have a strong grasp on the basic truths of Scripture. But the Bible is not just to be intellectually grasped and understood; it is to be obeyed. Knowledge without obedience can lead to deception. And finally, a life of love is the goal of Christianity. Paul said, "The goal of our instruction is love. . . . Some men, straying from these things, have turned aside to fruitless discussion" (1 Tim. 1:5,6).

Therefore, live a life that is characterized by believing God's truth and obeying His commands, but motivated by a pure and godly love.

Why do you feel cults have increased in number so much in our age?

How can you keep yourself and your loved ones safe from them?

41. Leaping Over Walls

For by Thee I can run upon a troop; and by my God I can leap over a wall (Ps. 18:29).

Most marathon runners acknowledge the reality of an experience known as "hitting the wall"—feeling totally drained physically and emotionally. When that happens, some drop out of the race, while others finish the remaining miles on sheer willpower. Overcoming this "wall" requires extreme mental and physical discipline.

David did not have marathons in mind when he wrote about leaping over walls. He was thinking of even more difficult experiences. David had been anointed king while evil King Saul was still on the throne. For ten years he waited, resisting the temptation to kill Saul because he believed he should not lay a hand on God's anointed. God removed Saul in His own way, and the shepherd boy became the greatest king in Israel's history.

David was able to do the difficult thing of being a godly king. But with God's help, he was able to do the even more difficult thing of waiting quietly in the background for God's timing. His testimony was, "I waited patiently for the Lord; and He inclined to me, and heard my cry" (Ps. 40:1). Whether it was ruling or waiting, he found God adequate.

God may be requiring something difficult of you. He may be asking you to do something that, in your eyes, seems impossible. You feel that others are far more qualified for the task than you are. Yet the feeling persists that God wants you to do it. In recognizing the height of the wall before you and the weakness of your heart within you, you are tempted to turn away, declaring simply, "I can't."

But never say "I can't" when God says "You can." David realized that with God he could leap over walls. Paul realized that "when I am weak, then I am strong" (2 Cor. 12:10). When we recognize our weakness and insufficiency and cry out to God for help, we discover that His power is made perfect in weakness (2 Cor. 12:9).

The self-assured and proud will crash into the wall and collapse. The fearful and timid will turn away from the wall and retreat. But Christians can leap over the wall and accomplish things they never thought possible. Even those who consider themselves weak, slow, and lacking in gifts can experience great fulfillment and power in their lives.

All this is by design; it's the way God set it up from the beginning. "God has chosen the foolish things of the world to shame the wise, and God has chosen the weak things of the world to shame the things which are strong" (1 Cor. 1:27). As long as we remember that we are weak, then the strength of Christ will rest upon us.

What role in your life (parent, Sunday school teacher, supervisor, etc.) do you feel least adequate to fulfill?

How can you tap into the power of Christ in order to accomplish difficult tasks?

42. Hurry! Hurry!

With the coming of dawn, the angels urged Lot, saying, "Hurry! Take your wife and your two daughters who are here, or you will be swept away when the city is punished." When he hesitated, the men grasped his hand and the hands of his wife and of his two daughters and led them safely out of the city (Gen. 19:15,16 NIV).

The normal pace of the Christian life is a careful, steady effort—neither sprinting ahead or lagging behind. Certainly, a believer is to avoid hastiness and impulsive decisions. Yet there is a time to rush. The angels warned Lot to hurry out of the city of Sodom as fast as he could, before the judgment of God fell upon it. A follower of Christ is to run quickly to get away from any place where God's judgment is going to fall. The angel told Lot to gather his family and flee for his life, never looking back.

Lot had problems from the beginning. The Scriptures tell us that after he separated from Abraham he pitched his tent near Sodom, a wicked city filled with homosexuality and other sins. Lot chose to live near that place, finally moving into the city and becoming very comfortable there. He never partook of their sin, but he lived among then. How many today are seeking to get as close to sin as they can without indulging in it?

Lot had become so comfortable and accepting of the sinful lifestyles around him that he hesitated when the angel told him to leave. The angel had to grasp his hand and literally drag him out of the city to safety. What a sad bunch of runners they must have been as they moved from the plains toward the mountains, two angels dragging a worldly believer and his little family reluctantly to safety.

Lot's experience shows us why we are not to be conformed to the world or to love its sinful ways. Tragedy came to his family because he allowed himself, his wife, and his daughters to be exposed to sinful people and temptations.

Do you realize that even before the final "Day of Judgment" God sometimes sends judgment for sin?

From what places or habits do you need to "flee"?

43. The Fighting Spirit

Fight the good fight of faith (1 Tim. 6:12).

The fighting spirit. Every good athlete has it. It's more than just the competitive urge. It's the drive to overcome obstacles and unwillingness to be kept down by difficulties or defeats. Some seem to have it, while others don't. Yet it can and must be developed!

A Hungarian target shooter used the skill and precision of his right arm to win the gold medal in the 1952 Olympics. Shortly after, he lost his right arm in a car accident. For three and a half years he practiced shooting at the target with his left arm. In 1956, at the Melbourne Olympics, he won his second gold medal in target shooting! The fighting spirit!

We see life either as a playground or a battlefield. If we are just out to enjoy ourselves, we will be defeated by the first conflicts that come into our lives. But if we recognize that life itself is a battlefield, then we will be prepared for whatever comes.

At the end of his life, the great apostle Paul declared triumphantly, "I have fought the good fight" (2 Tim. 4:7). To young Timothy, just beginning his spiritual life, Paul exhorted, "Fight the good fight" (1 Tim. 6:12). He also urged Timothy, "Suffer hardship with me, as a good soldier of Christ Jesus" (2 Tim. 2:3). This is the biblical view of life and faith: a battle, a warfare, a conflict with an enemy who is to be fought and defeated.

Who is the enemy? What is the nature of this battle?

We may be attacked in a variety of ways. It may be that some rejection or condemnation from other people has left us wounded. Perhaps in some area of our lives we have experienced repeated failures that have left us discouraged. Maybe evil thoughts have left us fearful, or a series of reversals and setbacks have left us confused. Behind all of these attacks lie one of two enemies.

The first enemy is Satan, who wants to destroy us. His final defeat is sure, but for the present he can still do us harm. Therefore, we must be alert to his schemes and take our stand against him. When we resist him, he must flee from us, according to James 4:7. One way to resist him is by prayer in the powerful name of the Lord Jesus Christ.

The other enemy we must battle is the flesh, or our old sinful natures. In many ways, this is the worst of the two enemies because the flesh dwells within us. We don't have control over the hurts and reversals that come into our lives, but we do have control over our reactions to them. Paul wrote, "If you are living according to the flesh, you must die; but if by the Spirit you are putting to death the deeds of the body, you will live" (Rom. 8:13). As Christians, there is a great conflict going on in our hearts between our sinful natures and our new natures. (see Gal. 5:16–18). But through the Spirit we can fight the good fight and win this battle.

Many would agree that life is a battlefield, but they feel they have been defeated forever. It's at this very point that Paul exhorts us to rise to our feet and fight the battle. Many have found the following statement a motivational turning point in their lives: "Begin a war you expect to win and plan on many battles." We recognize that some battles may be lost in the process of the conflict, but each loss will only give us new determination to fight on and win the war.

As we maintain this fighting spirit we will some day be able to say with Paul, "I have fought the good fight, I have finished the course, I have kept the faith; in the future there is laid up for me the crown of righteousness" (2 Tim. 4:7,8).

What battles are you presently facing?

What must you do to fight the good fight?

44. Running Toward
the Enemy

Then it happened that when the Philistine rose and came and drew near to meet David, that David ran quickly toward the battle line to meet the Philistine. And David put his hand into his bag and took from it a stone and slung it, and struck the Philistine on his forehead (1 Sam. 17:48,49).

We are all familiar with the story of David and Goliath. The courage of this young shepherd boy, probably a teen-ager, was a great contrast to the weakness of the whole Israelite army. No one else but David was willing to face the enemy. He not only met the enemy head on, but he ran to the battle line! This was no slow trot; he literally sprinted to meet the challenge.

Why did David have this courage when everyone else wanted to run in the other direction? How could he have such confidence with only a sling and five smooth stones, when the soldiers with their swords and shields were trembling in their boots?

Read David's own words: "Your servant was tending his father's sheep. When a lion or a bear came and took a lamb from the flock, I went out after him and attacked him. . . . The LORD who delivered me from the paw of the lion and from the paw of the bear, He will deliver me from the hand of this Philistine" (1 Sam. 17:34,37). David had seen God's deliverance in smaller matters, and rightly concluded from his experience that God would be able to deliver him from the greater enemy. If God could handle bears and lions, God could handle a Philistine—even a giant one.

The instant David won the battle, another battle began. It was as if a starter's gun had gone off at the beginning of a ten-kilometer run with two thousand runners. "When the Philistines saw that their champion was dead, they fled" (1 Sam. 17:51). The Israelites pursued the Philistines and destroyed them. David's personal victory over Goliath led the Israelites to a national victory over the Philistines. That great victory over an army wouldn't have happened if there had not been the victory over a giant, and that victory wouldn't have happened if there hadn't been victory over bears and lions.

When a man or woman is facing a battle, small or great, it must be faced squarely if future victories are to be won. We can run away from the battle line—or toward it, as David did. We may feel ill-equipped, but if we know we are on God's side and He is our deliverance, who can stand against us?

What giants or enemies are there in your life that must be faced squarely?

Can you remember any past deliverances God has given you that would strengthen your confidence for this present conflict?

45. A Father's Run

*When he came to his senses, he said, "How many of my
father's hired men have more than enough bread, but I am
dying here with hunger! I will get up and go to my father,
and will say to him, 'Father, I have sinned against
heaven, and in your sight; I am no longer worthy to be
called your son; make me as one of your hired men.' "
And he got up and came to his father. But while he was
still a long way off, his father saw him, and felt compassion for him, and ran and embraced him, and kissed him
(Luke 15:17–20).*

Early one Thanksgiving morning, my ten-year-old son and
I ran in a five-mile race called the "Turkey Trot." This was
Peter's first five-mile race. Although there was a combination
of snow and rain falling, he had an excellent time, and in the
last hundred yards he courageously beat out another boy
about his age. A friend of ours who is a dedicated and gifted
distance runner took first place. After receiving the trophy, he
immediately walked over and handed it to my son, saying,
"Take this trophy. You deserve it more than I do." A wide
smile appeared on Peter's face as he carried the treasure home
to show Mom.

Jesus Christ gives us the trophy of His righteousness,
which allows us to enter heaven. We could never earn heaven
on our own merits; it is given to us out of grace as a free gift.
In the same way, the son in Jesus' parable did not earn his
father's love and forgiveness. What he deserved was judgment and rejection. Yet, out of grace, the father welcomed
and received him back. In fact, while the son was still a long
way off, the father saw him and ran to embrace him. So, too,
our heavenly Father runs to meet anyone who returns to Him.

Every Christian has been embraced in love and forgiveness by his heavenly Father. Yet many believers still feel a sense of condemnation when they think about their relationship with God. They feel rejected and cast off by a God who seems very distant. But the truth of the matter is that every repentant believer has the arms of his heavenly Father encircling and tightly embracing him in total acceptance. No judgment or rejection remains for the person who has, like the Prodigal Son, returned home repentant and humble. As Paul wrote, "There is therefore now no condemnation for those who are in Christ Jesus" (Rom. 8:1).

Visualize this father running down the road toward his defeated son, who is returning home in humiliation. Picture the embrace, the kiss, the tears of joy. Picture the son only getting halfway through his prepared confession before the father interrupts him. Picture the robe and the ring and the sandals, provided at the father's request. Picture the feast and the celebration that followed.

This is the extent to which God receives and accepts those who return home to Him. Not only is there "no condemnation," but there is full sonship established. And with sonship comes the robe of Christ's righteousness, the ring of spiritual authority, the sandals that cover the feet of those who bring glad tidings and the celebration and joy of feasting on the Father's food in the Father's house. This is the inheritance and blessing of every true child of God.

Do you visualize God as your Judge or as your loving heavenly Father?

How can you use the truth of Romans 8:1 to overcome feelings of condemnation?

46. Thirsty

If any man is thirsty, let him come to Me and drink. He who believes in Me, as the Scripture said, "From his innermost being shall flow rivers of living water" (John 7:37,38).

A person who runs a long race, such as a marathon, needs to drink water during the race. A runner's body loses water through perspiration and respiration, and if it's not replaced the person will dehydrate and experience muscle cramps. Therefore, race organizers set up stations along the course of the race and offer the runners water as they go by.

We also experience a spiritual thirst. Only Jesus Christ can satisfy this thirst. He says, "Come to Me and drink." He is the rock from which the Israelites drank in the Old Testament (see Ex. 17:6; 1 Cor. 10:1–4). In the New Testament, He is the One who promises water that would satisfy eternally (see John 4:13,14). He is the One who gives not just a drop or a trickle, but streams of living water. He is the only source of spiritual satisfaction and fulfillment. He is the fountainhead from which the water of the Spirit abundantly flows.

D. L. Moody said the trouble with Christians is that they are leaky vessels. We've received the water of life, but we have a tendency to dry up. What is the cause of this spiritual dryness?

God has established the spiritual life in such a way that a one-time decision to accept Christ will not provide ongoing satisfaction. You can't drink a gallon of water on the first day of the month and hope to make it the next thirty days without a drink. It's God's desire that once we've come to Christ for salvation, we keep coming to Him for satisfaction. This is a daily, even moment-by-moment, experience.

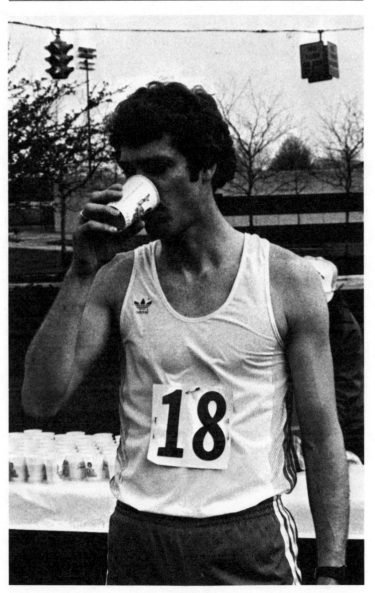

Sometimes we turn to other sources to find satisfaction, even though we know we can find it only in Christ. God said, through Jeremiah, "My people have committed two evils: They have forsaken Me, the Fountain of living waters, to hew for themselves cisterns, broken cisterns, that can hold no water" (Jer. 2:13). The Israelites were forsaking God and turning to idols that could never satisfy their spiritual thirst.

Many Christians build their own "broken cisterns." Some look to a particular relationship or to their church for satisfaction. Others seek it in sports, or television, or food. Still others pursue success, or fame, or prosperity. Many of these are legitimate pleasures, but they can never give ultimate satisfaction or fulfillment.

Each time we feel ourselves drying up we are to run to Christ. Even as the race organizers offer water to the runners, so Christ freely offers the fresh flowing waters of the Spirit (see Is. 55:1). As we trust Christ and obey His Word, He will come to us with refreshment and blessing.

When was the last time you were spiritually dry?

What "broken cisterns" have you constructed rather than turning to Christ for refreshment?

47. The Most Exciting Run

The angel answered and said to the women, "Do not be afraid; for I know that you are looking for Jesus who has been crucified. He is not here, for He has risen, just as He said. Come, see the place where He was lying. And go quickly and tell His disciples that He has risen from the dead; and behold, He is going before you into Galilee, there you will see Him; behold, I have told you." And they departed quickly from the tomb with fear and great joy and ran to report it to His disciples (Matt. 28:5–8).

There was a time when the experts considered the four-minute mile an unbreakable barrier. They believed that at that speed the human body would run out of oxygen at a certain point near four minutes. Think of the tremendous excitement there must have been on May 6, 1954, when Roger Bannister ran his history-making, record-smashing 3.59.4 mile.

Yet the most exciting run in human history set no world records. There were no famous athletes involved and their time was not even clocked. The runners were women (both named Mary), who discovered that Jesus' tomb was empty and that He was alive. Out of fear, joy, and pure excitement they ran to tell the disciples that Jesus had risen from the dead, as He had claimed He would.

After Christ's death there must have been much depression among His followers. Their hopes were smashed and their leader was publicly humiliated and crucified. What was there to look forward to? Then came the Resurrection! For three days these women had been walking around with their heads hanging. Suddenly they find themselves racing down the road with joy.

When the apostle Paul was under great pressure, facing one

of the gravest trials of his life, he too found hope in the Resurrection. "We were burdened excessively, beyond our strength, so that we despaired even of life. . . in order that we should not trust in ourselves, but in God who raises the dead" (2 Cor. 1:8,9). Only a religion that can make something dead alive again is able to help people overcome despair. Christianity is the only religion whose founder and leader is still alive!

A popular Christian song says, "Because He lives, I can face tomorrow." If Jesus Christ overcame death, He can overcome any problem I may face. He can even take a situation or relationship that has died and bring it to life again. That is resurrection power!

Are there any situations or relationships in your life that have become so bad that the word "dead" could be applied?

How can the resurrection power of Christ bring you new hope and victory?

48. Looking Back

One thing I do: forgetting what lies behind and reaching forward to what lies ahead, I press on toward the goal for the prize of the upward call of God in Christ Jesus (Phil. 3:13,14).

Looking back can be dangerous for a runner. In the late 1950s, Roger Bannister and John Landy ran against each other in what was billed as the "Dream Mile." The whole world focused on this race between two of the premier milers of the decade. Both men were capable of setting a new world record, under four minutes. The first lap was a little sluggish, but the runners were still within reach of a record-breaking time. As the race continued, Bannister began to fall behind. Going around the last curve on the last lap, Landy looked back over his left shoulder to see where his opponent was. At that very instant Bannister, who had caught up with Landy and was just to his right, shot ahead of Landy. By the time Landy looked forward again, Bannister had opened a one-yard lead, which he kept for the final one hundred yards to the finish line. By looking back, John Landy had lost the race of the century.

Looking back can be dangerous spiritually also. The Christian is not to dwell on his past, lest he become discouraged. Always his attention is to be straight ahead toward his goal: Jesus Christ.

Lot's wife looked back and was turned into a pillar of salt. Jesus warned that, "No one, after putting his hand to the plow and looking back, is fit for the kingdom of God" (Luke 9:62). Focusing on past failures is a common temptation. Often we mentally relive a bad experience over and over again. Satan can do this kind of work on the screens of our minds. He is called the "accuser of our brethren . . . who accuses them before our God day and night. And they overcame him because of the blood of the Lamb" (Rev. 12:10,11). The accusations may be true, but if we are Christians then the slate has been wiped clean by the blood of Christ.

Paul said he forgot what was behind. How does one accomplish this? We are told that the mind is like a computer, with everything safely stored away but easily recallable at any time. "Forgetting" does not mean we somehow become absent-minded. Rather, it means that we choose not to focus on the past.

Some fifteen years ago, I was a teacher and track coach in the inner city. I have some painful memories connected with this year of teaching, and they can be recalled in full detail at any time. But by the grace of God, I have been able to choose not to dwell upon these memories each time they arise.

Looking back not only discourages a person, but it takes his gaze off of Jesus Christ—the goal of his life. The door to the past must be shut if we are to make any progress. Forget what is behind and strain forward toward what is ahead!

List the negative consequences of dwelling on past failures.

Develop a strategy for choosing to think about Christ whenever old negative memories arise.

49. Don't Run Alone

I will ask the Father, and He will give you another Helper, that He may be with you forever; that is the Spirit of truth" (John 14:16,17).

Each year my dad and I run in a five-mile race on Thanksgiving morning. A good friend of ours, Bill Long, also runs in this race. Bill has made the qualifying time for the Olympic tryouts in the marathon, so this race is just a light workout for him. Each year he wins the trophy for the fastest runner, and my dad wins the trophy for the oldest runner. Bill's usual procedure is to win the race and then jog back and meet Dad and run beside him to give him some encouragement during the final mile or so of the race.

In many ways, Bill's practice of winning and then returning to accompany and encourage other runners reminds us of the Lord Jesus. Christ ran victoriously by living a perfect life. Then, having died for our sins, He rose from the dead and ascended into heaven. Through His Spirit He has returned to earth to be with us, running alongside each Christian to encourage him in his race of faith.

The Greek word translated "Helper" in John 14:16 is *paraklētos*. It means "to come alongside of," as when one ship comes alongside another ship in distress to give it aid. So the Holy Spirit comes alongside us to encourage and exhort us.

Women are warned never to run outside alone because of the danger of being attacked. This danger can usually be eliminated by the presence of another person running at her side. It is the same in the spiritual race of life. "Your adversary, the devil, prowls around like a roaring lion, seeking someone to devour" (1 Pet. 5:8).

In contrast is the continual help of the Holy Spirit. "There is a friend who sticks closer than a brother" (Prov. 18:24). This Friend is not only close to us, but He is also powerful within our hearts. "Greater is He who is in you than he who is in the world" (1 John 4:4). The Holy Spirit, who indwells each believer, is more powerful than Satan and all his demons. Therefore, as Christians we need not live our lives in fear but in confident trust in the presence and power of our Friend who runs beside us and lives within us.

Another way to overcome the loneliness of life is to find a prayer partner. Homemakers, businessmen, students—people from all walks of life have found the practice of meeting regularly with their prayer partner a great blessing. Some have even practiced this while living in different cities. A fifteen-minute call once a week to share a time of prayer is not expensive compared to the benefits received. The presence of the Spirit in our lives is very real, yet sometimes we need to hear the human voice of a friend who says, "I'll pray for you." It is often through a prayer partner that the Spirit's constant presence and help becomes real to us.

Where does the Holy Spirit dwell?

How can you be sure you are not running your race alone?

50. The Running Boom

And the things which you have heard from me in the presence of many witnesses, these entrust to faithful men, who will be able to teach others (2 Tim. 2:2).

Few sports have caught on like running. Today, millions are out running on the streets and paths of our country. Why? What was their motivation for overcoming the sedentary life? Were they manipulated by a massive publicity campaign? Were there thousands of hours of TV coverage of marathons and road races? Were leaflets and tracts distributed to people as they left their offices?

The driving force behind the running movement is found in none of these things. Although now there are magazines devoted to the sport, and there is growing TV coverage, this was not the case in the beginning. I believe the secret to the growth of the movement was a grass-roots, person-to-person sharing of the benefits runners experienced. One person enthusiastically told a friend, who got involved and then repeated the process. Each person shared the successes and defeats he or she was experiencing. Workouts, shoes, injuries, and goals were all discussed freely with anyone who would listen. In spiritual terms, a one-to-one discipling movement took place.

Jesus said we are to go into the world and make disciples of all nations (see Matt. 28:19). The calling of every Christian is to win people to Christ and then to help them become His obedient followers. This takes much love, time, and effort, but a person who is discipled can become a disciple-maker. This strategy of multiplication is seen in the life of Jesus, the master disciple-maker. He started with twelve men who came to know Him intimately over a three-year period. During that time, Jesus encouraged, rebuked, taught, warned, and equipped these men, and after they received the Holy Spirit they were sent out to be His witnesses. Through these ordinary men, a worldwide spiritual movement began that will eventually fill heaven with thousands upon thousands from every race, tribe, nation, and people of the earth.

Someone has said that only two things will survive this world: the Word of God and people. If this is all that really matters, then isn't it worth the effort to pour your life into something of lasting value? Paul said, "Keep seeking the things above, where Christ is, seated at the right hand of God" (Col. 3:1). Building the Word of God into peoples' lives is of eternal value.

You don't have to be a super Christian with a dynamic personality to disciple someone. God uses ordinary people to accomplish His purposes. But ordinary people, once they realize they are part of a worldwide movement directed by Jesus Christ Himself, become motivated and enthusiastic to live for Him. Are you involved? Will you have something of eternal value to show for the brief years you spend on this planet? "Only one life, t'will soon be past, only what's done for Christ will last."

"Is your life counting for something of eternal significance?"

Whom could you begin meeting with on a weekly basis to encourage toward maturity in Christ?

51. Finishing the Race

I have fought the good fight, I have finished the race, I have kept the faith. Finally, there is laid up for me the crown of righteousness, which the Lord, the righteous Judge, will give me on that Day; and not to me only, but also to all who have loved His appearing (2 Tim. 4:7,8 NKJB).

It has been estimated that 25 percent of all marathon runners never finish any given race. It's such a grueling test of strength and will that just to cross the finish line is a great achievement.

Many people find their lives are the same type of grueling test. And with the rapid pace of our society, its changing values, and increased pressure and stress, many drop out of the race.

The Christian life is much like a marathon. There are many who seem to begin well but who finish poorly or not at all. Saul, the first king of Israel, was a promising and humble young man. Yet he rebelled against God and is now considered one of Israel's worst kings. Demas, in the New Testament, was one of Paul's effective helpers. But he forsook Paul in a time of crisis, and he is remembered as one who abandoned the work of God for worldliness.

Head and shoulders above them all stands the apostle Paul. In his final days he wrote from a prison in Rome: "I have finished the race." From the time he began the race until the end of his days, he was faithful—not ashamed of Christ but testifying boldly for Him. We need to follow his example and be finishers in the race that is set before us.

John Kelly, at age seventy-three, crossed the finish line of the 1981 Boston marathon to the loudest and longest applause

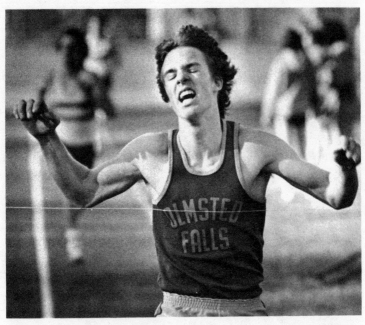

received by anyone other than the winners. But the applause wasn't primarily because of his age; rather, it was because he had just completed his fiftieth Boston marathon! John Kelly is a finisher!

The apostle Paul won the crown of righteousness because he finished well. That crown is awaiting all who are finishers. To finish the race means to be fully obedient to Christ all the days of my life. It means to humbly follow Christ and stay within the boundary lines He has set for me. It means to continue growing in purity of heart until the day I see Him face to face and become fully like Him (see 1 John 3:2,3). To finish the race means that I give myself fully to the work He has assigned me so that when my life is done I can say, along with Jesus, "I glorified Thee on the earth, having accomplished the work which Thou hast given Me to do" (John 17:4).

It would seem that Satan's primary attack upon the church today is in the area of the family. Even the marriages of some well-known Christian leaders are breaking up. The divorce rate of believers is approaching that of unbelievers. The world looks on and sees little difference between itself and the church. Many Christians are not finishing well.

But the power of Christ is available to counteract the pressures of this rebellious generation. Even where there has been failure, God is able to pick up the pieces, grant forgiveness, and give new purpose and power for living. The promise of Christ remains true: "He who overcomes, and he who keeps My deeds until the end, TO HIM I WILL GIVE AUTHORITY OVER THE NATIONS" (Rev. 2:26).

Commit yourself now to the way of endurance and overcoming. Like Paul, be a finisher.

Are you contemplating any course of action that would bring disgrace to the name of Christ?

Is your love for Christ getting warmer each day or has it begun to cool off?

52. The Prize

Do you not know that those who run in a race all run,
but only one receives the prize? Run in such a way that
you may win. . . . I press on toward the goal for the prize
. . . (1 Cor. 9:24; Phil. 3:14).

Runners have received all sorts of prizes for their efforts over the years—ribbons, trophies, medals, and plaques. In more recent times, competitors have received everything from toilet kits to perfume. Some runners could open their own T-shirt stores! Successful runners enjoy the double rewards of fame and fortune. Whether the prize is something as small as a ribbon, as great as an Olympic gold medal, or as intangible as a feeling of knowing you did your best, everyone loves to receive rewards.

The concept of rewards is built into the very fabric of life. This is true in the spiritual realm as well as the natural. The Scriptures say, "He who comes to God must believe that He is, and that He is a rewarder of those who seek Him" (Heb. 11:6). Some of these rewards will come in heaven, but others can be experienced in this life.

Although a Christian is not immune from the trials of life that come to everyone, he has access to a better quality of life than an unbeliever. He can have real peace of mind, a deep inner joy, and a sense of fulfillment and purpose in life. Within the body of Christ, he will experience close and beautiful friendships that would not otherwise have been possible. David encouraged others to praise the Lord and "forget none of His benefits" (Ps. 103:2).

There are also heavenly rewards for those who have run faithfully. The apostle Paul spoke of laboring for an "imperishable wreath," and waiting to receive the "crown of righ-

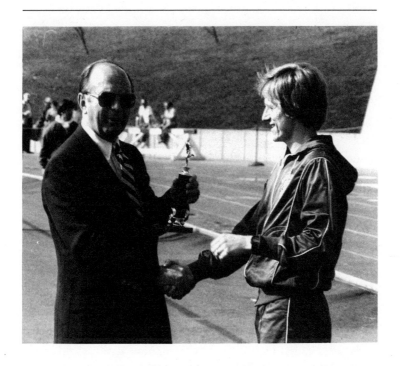

teousness" (1 Cor. 9:25; 2 Tim. 4:8). We do not know exactly what the nature of these rewards are, but the Scriptures give us a glimpse of a prize even greater than these eternal rewards—Jesus Christ Himself! Every other reward will pale in significance when we see our Lord and Savior face to face.

The apostle Paul wrote, "I count all things to be loss in view of the surpassing value of knowing Jesus Christ my Lord" (Phil. 3:8). This is the greatest of all prizes!

Knowing Jesus Christ is not something we must wait for until we get to heaven. Our relationship with Him begins in this life as we put our faith in Christ and take Him to be our spiritual coach. He is the best coach a person could desire. He has set the example for us with His sinless life. He has called us from the ranks of the spectators and made us participants in the spiritual run. He has entered us in the race of faith and even paid the entrance fee for us with His own blood and righteousness. What coach has ever gone this far for his runners?

Christ has enrolled us in His classroom and is teaching us the rules of the race. He warns us of the narrowness and length of the course and of the dangers of disqualification. He shows us vivid pictures of some of His people's victories and failures—people like David, Joseph, John, Mary, Jonah, and Elijah.

Christ has taken us into His gymnasium and is training us through a disciplined spiritual fitness program personally designed for each individual. He teaches us the importance of hard work as well as the restfulness of faith. He trains us not to look at the other runners, but to keep our eyes focused on Him. He helps us to be consistent in spiritual muscle-building by spending time in His word and prayer each day. He gives us our uniform to wear—the shoes of the gospel and the garments of salvation.

Finally, Christ leads us into competition to be tested in the trials of life. He is able to keep us from falling, and when we do fall He quickly lifts us up. He is able to heal all our injuries; the ones He doesn't heal He uses to mature and humble us. When we "hit the wall" He restores and refreshes us, quenching our thirst with the water of His Spirit. He leads the way, sets the pace, runs beside us, and even indwells us. He lives in us and through us so that we can run and not grow weary; He enables us to finish the race well. He is the author and perfecter of our faith, the one who starts us off in this run of faith and who will ultimately carry us successfully across the finish line by His mighty strength.

The person who has come into a personal relationship with Jesus Christ has already received the richest and greatest prize possible. If we know Christ we can desire nothing more, yet we grow richer each day. A personal relationship with the living God is far different from a trophy—it is a dynamic, growing, developing reality. In short, Jesus Christ *is* the prize!

List some of the benefits or rewards you have experienced because of following Christ.

Meditate on Jesus Christ as the ultimate prize.

Kenneth P. Radke, a former physical education teacher and track coach, earned his B.S. degree at Bowling Green State University and his M.E. degree at Kent State University. He served five years on the staff of Inter-Varsity Christian Fellowship and, for the past nine years, has been assistant pastor at Grace Christian and Missionary Alliance Church in Middleburg Heights, Ohio.